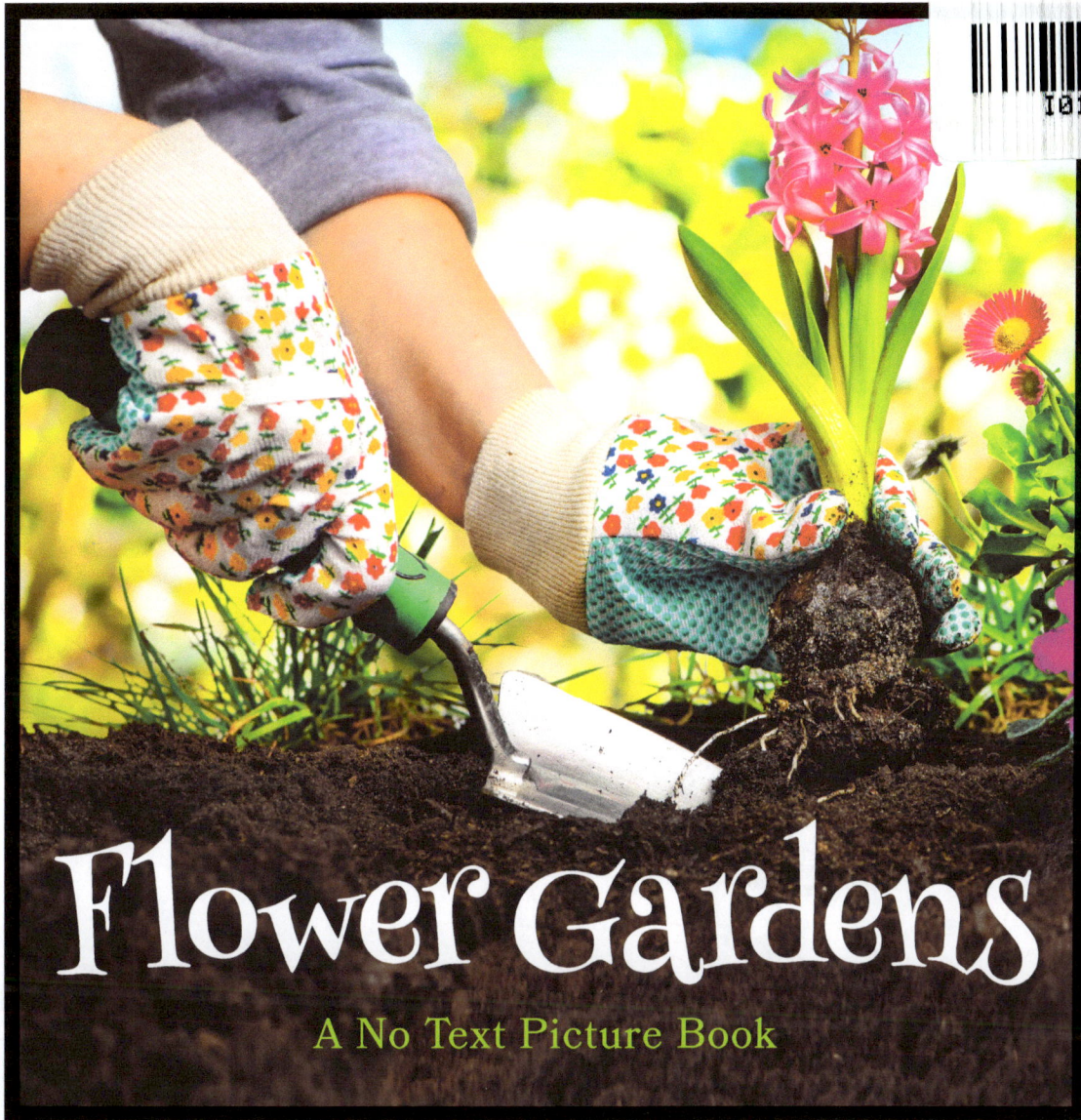

Flower Gardens

A No Text Picture Book

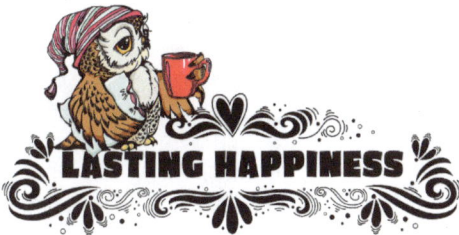

Lasting Happiness

ISBN: 978-1-990181-24-5

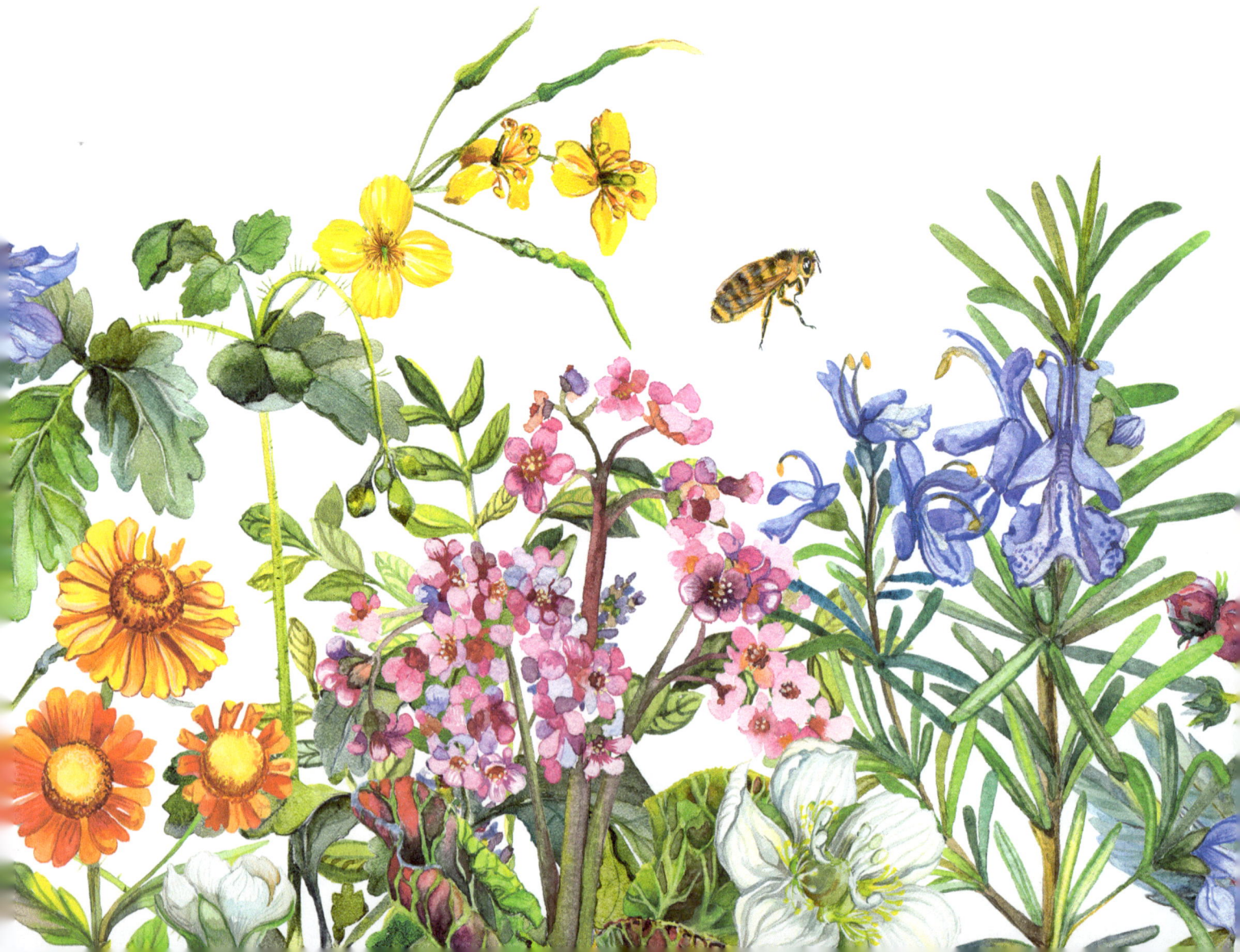

To:

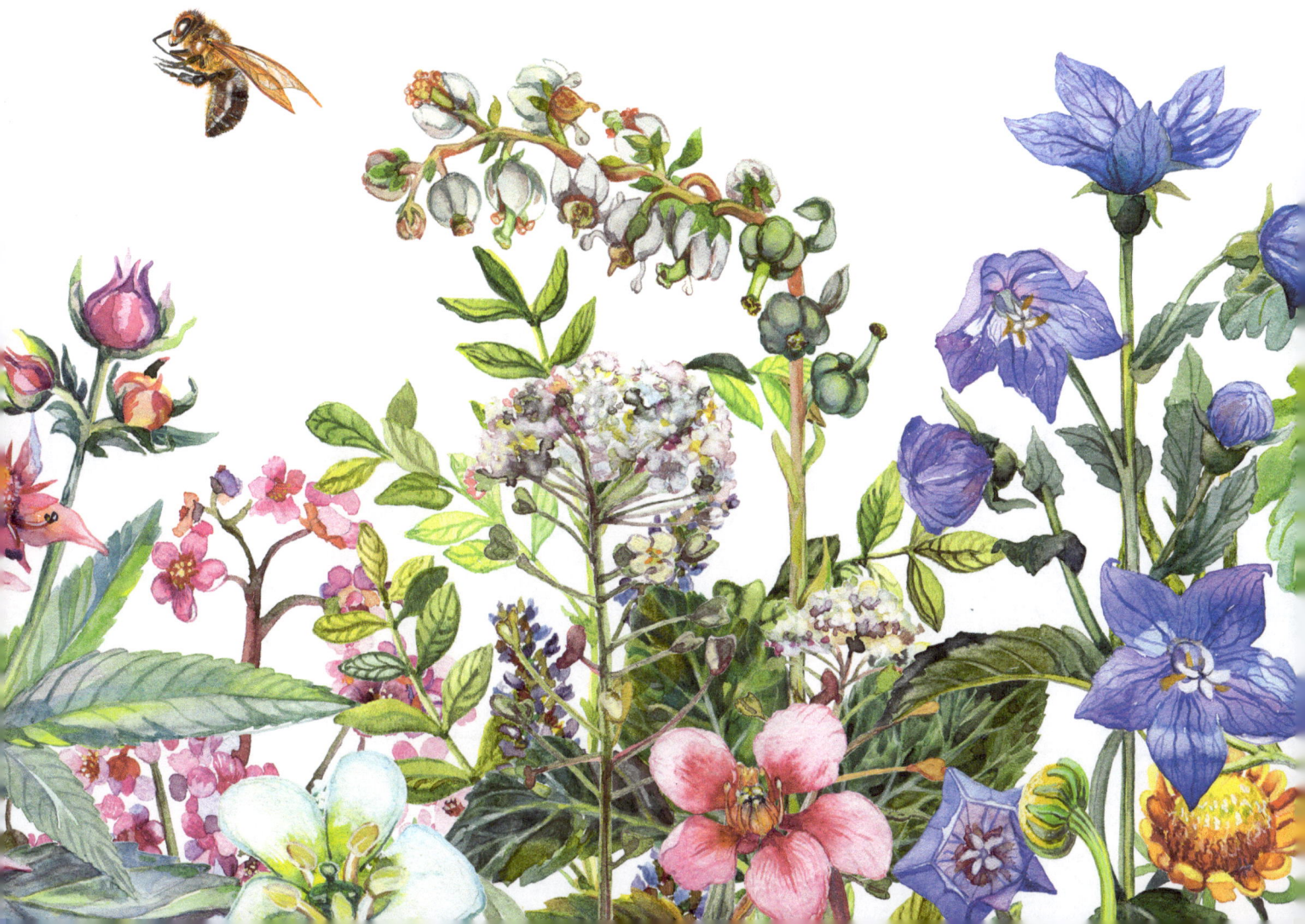

FROM:

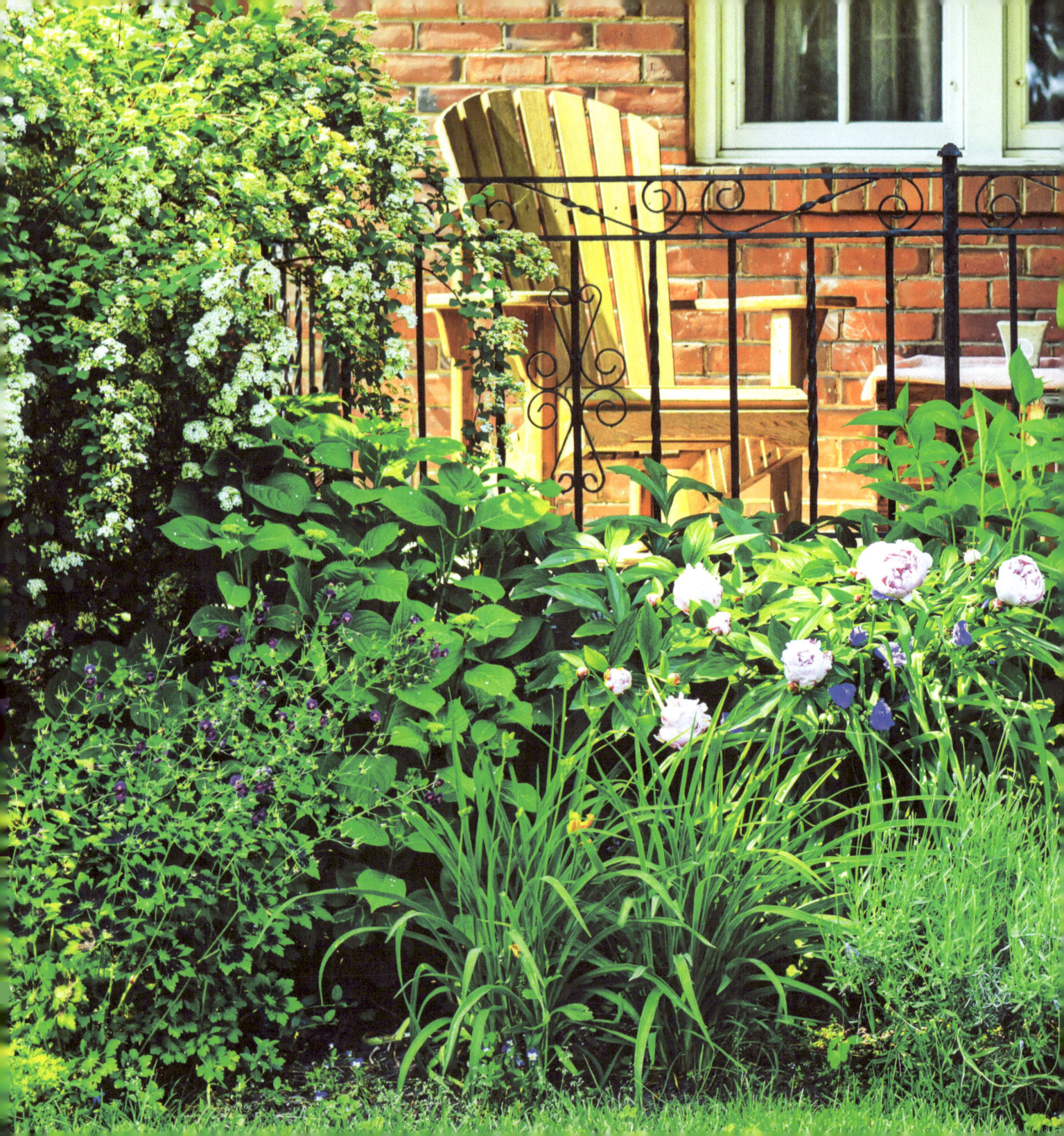

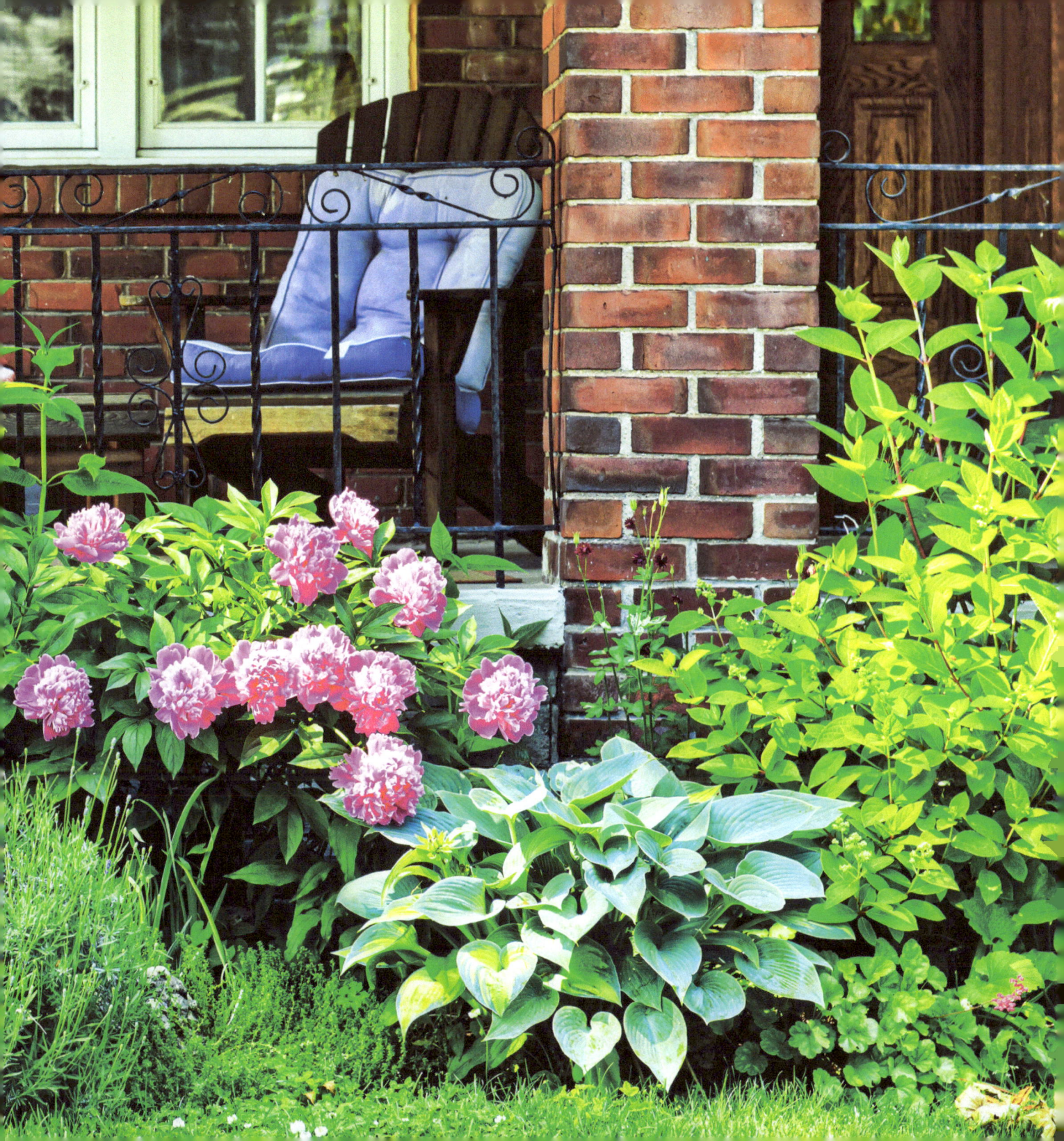

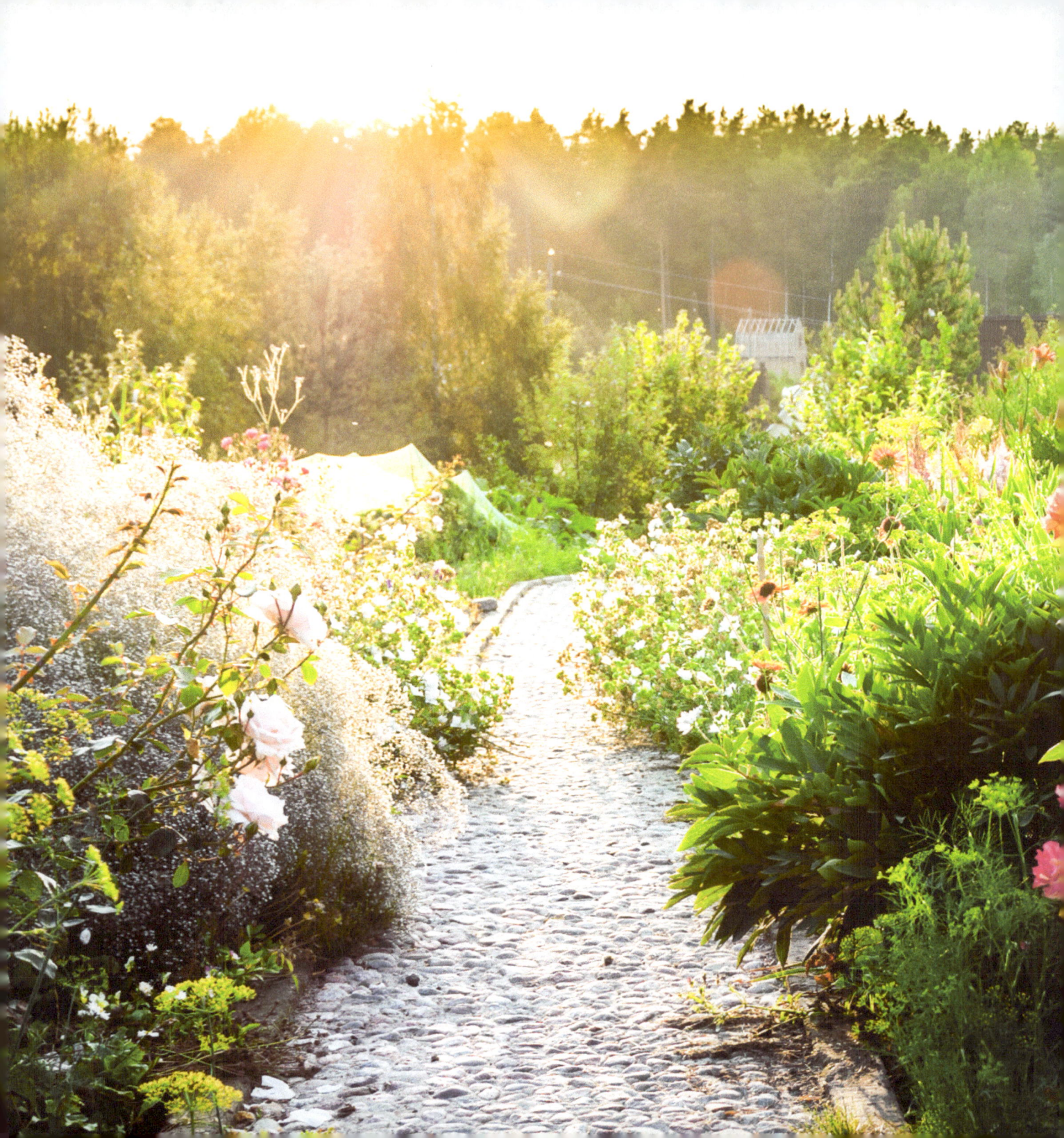

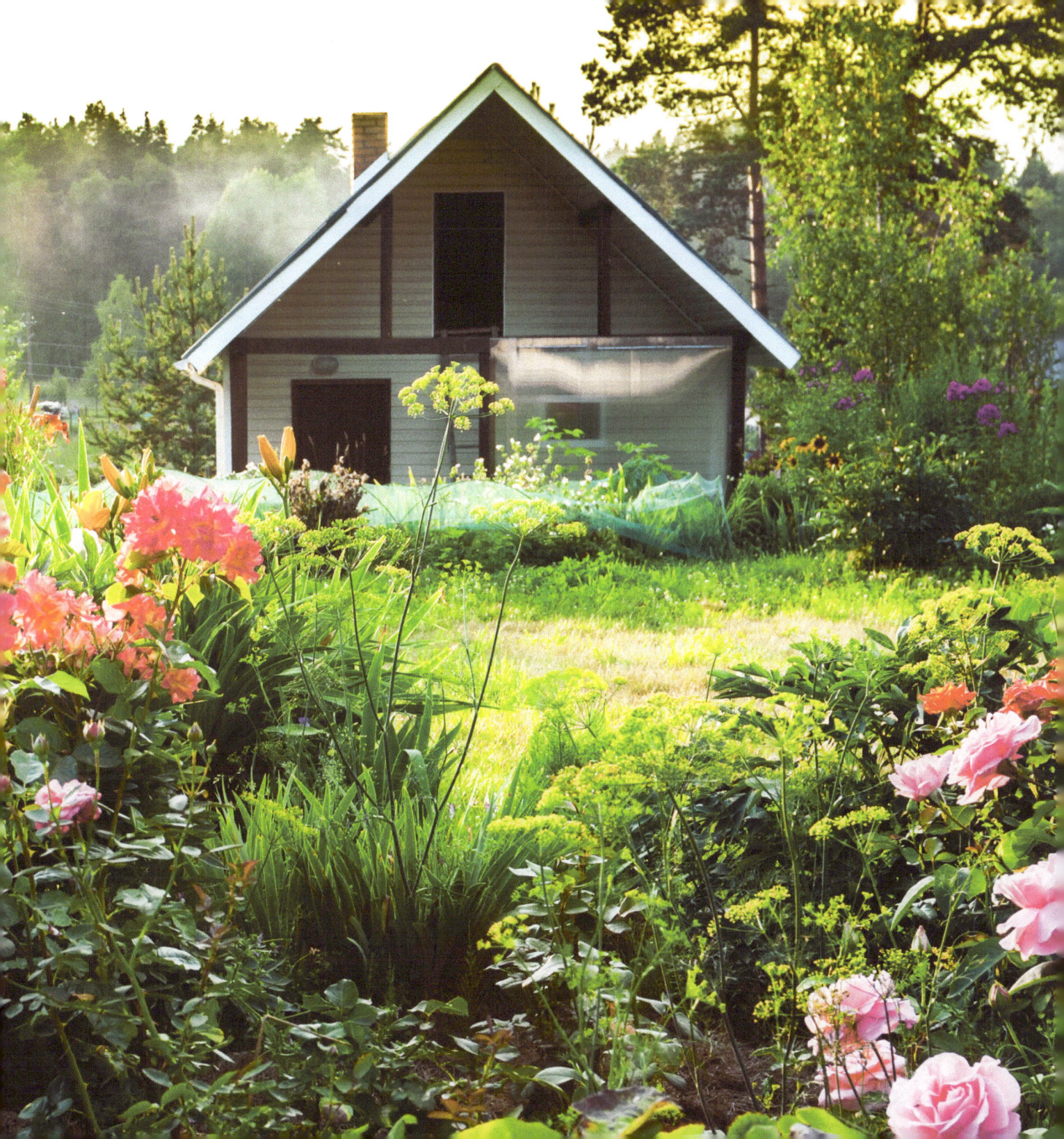

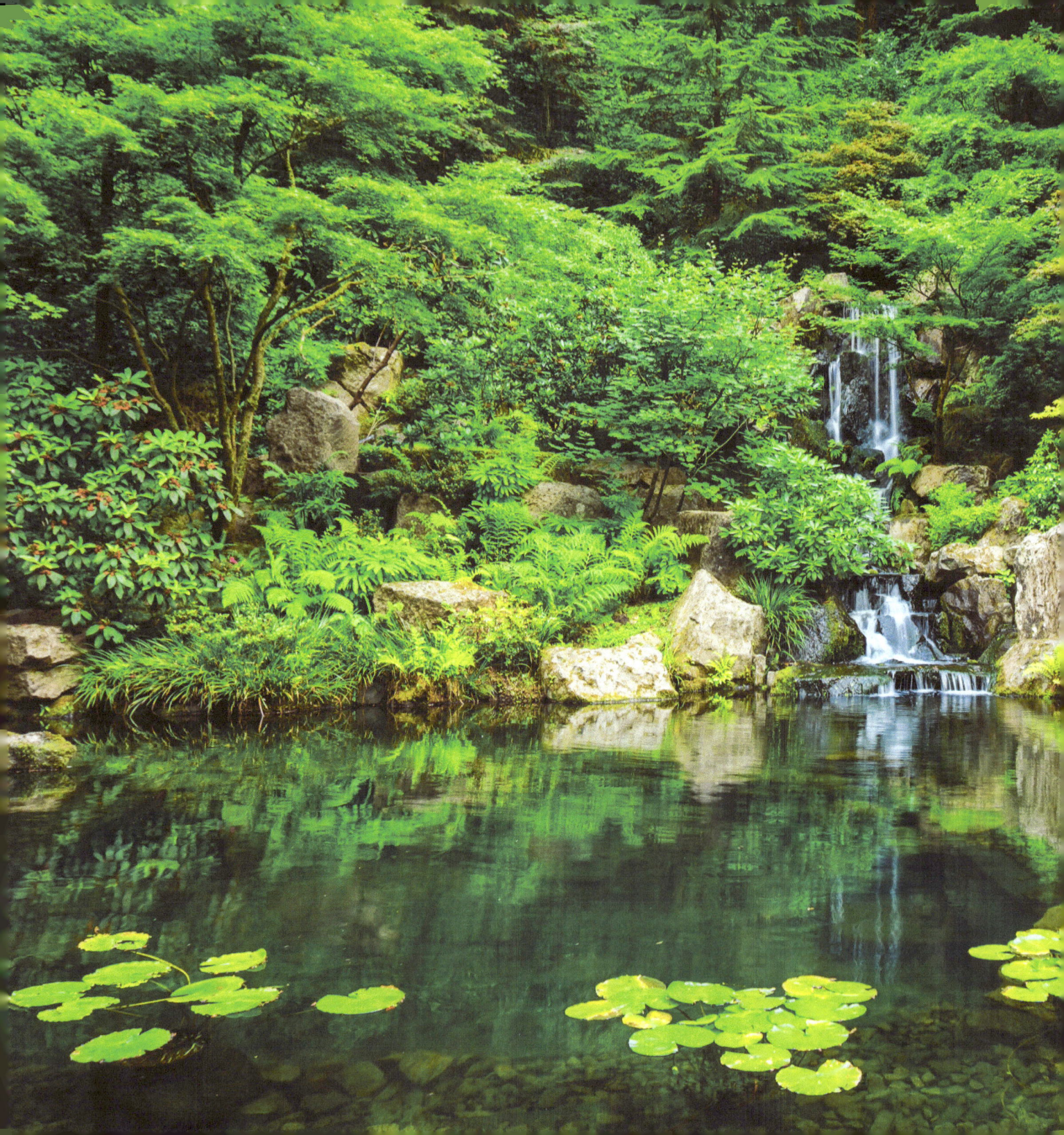

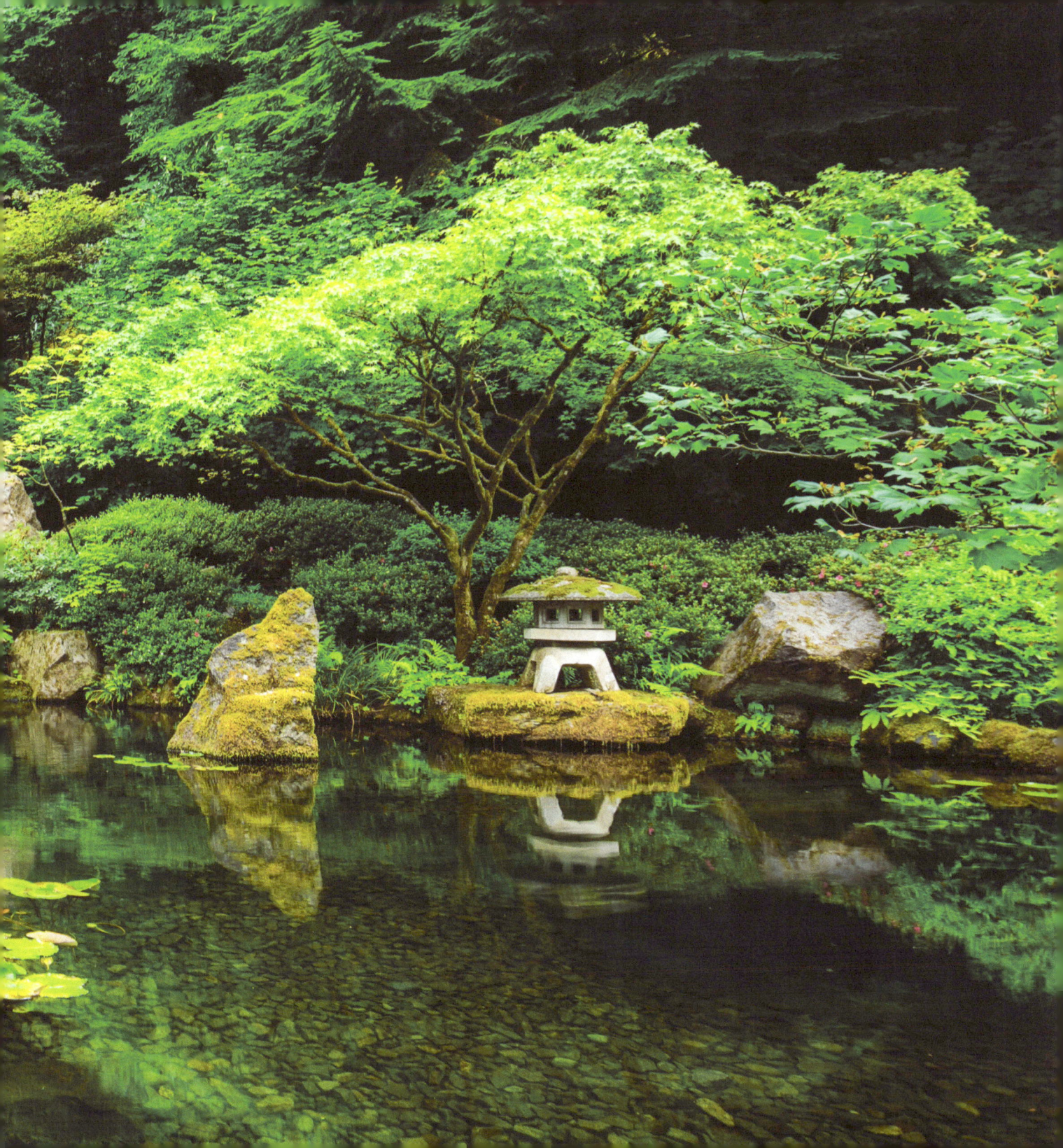

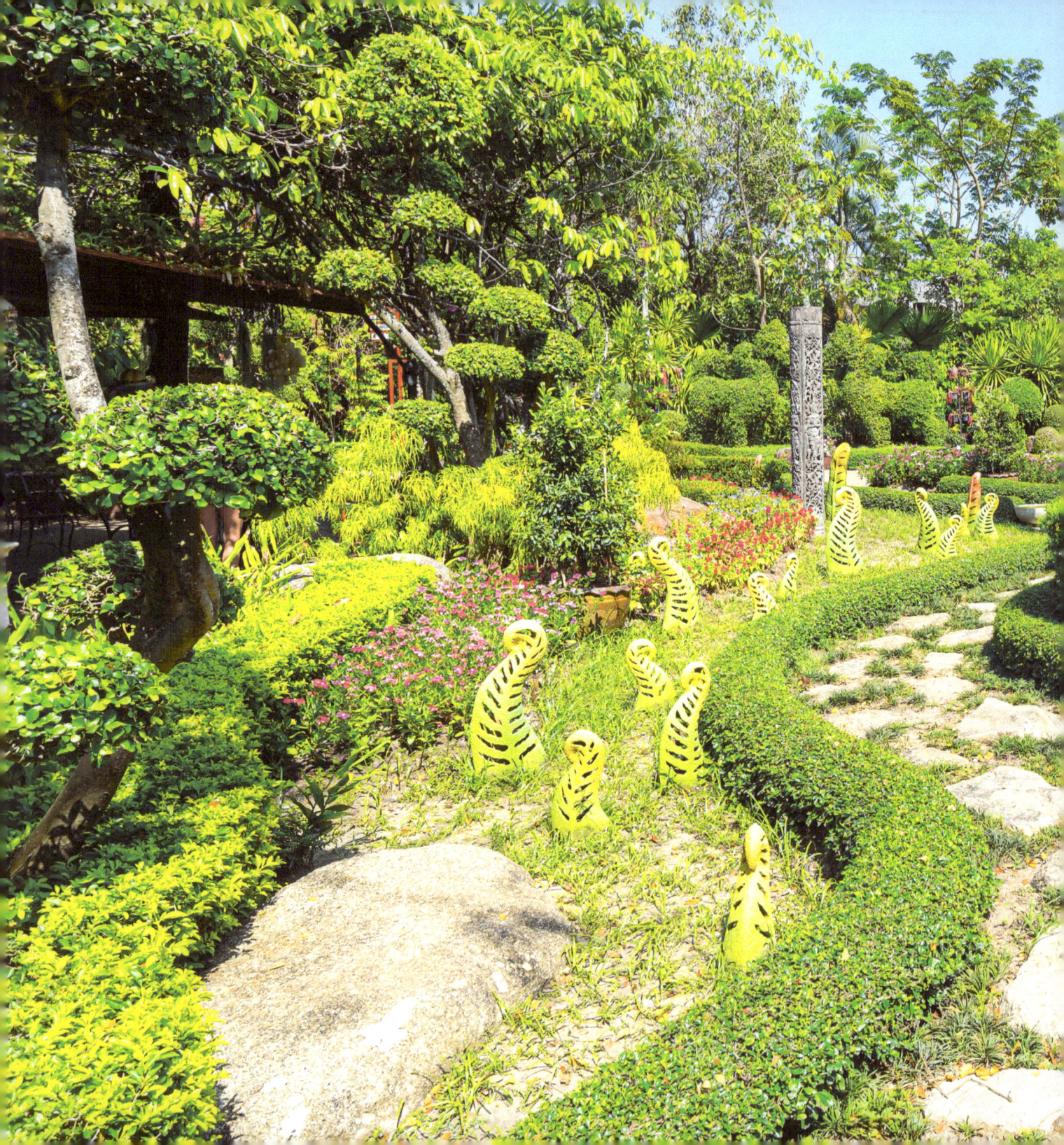

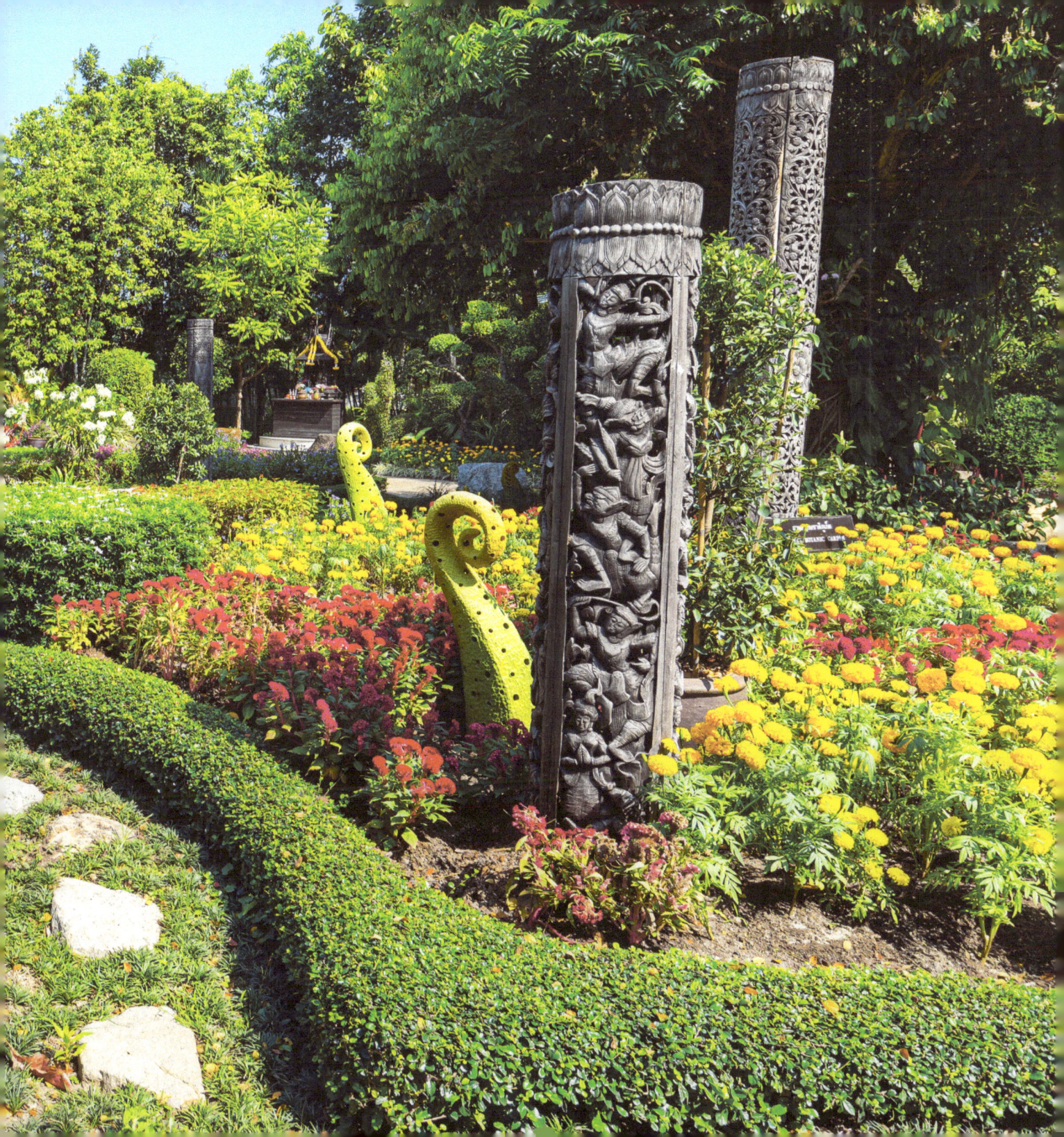

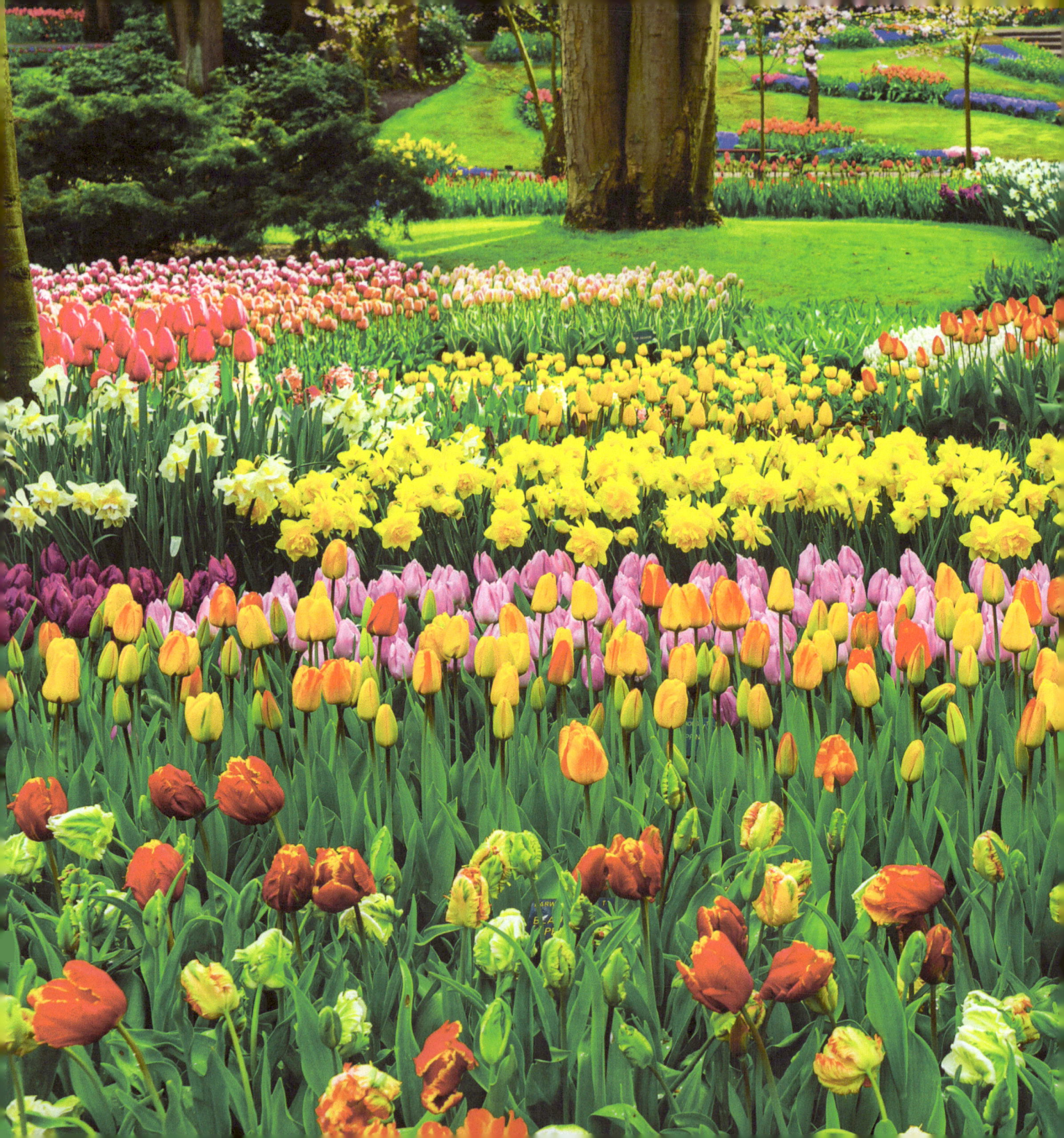

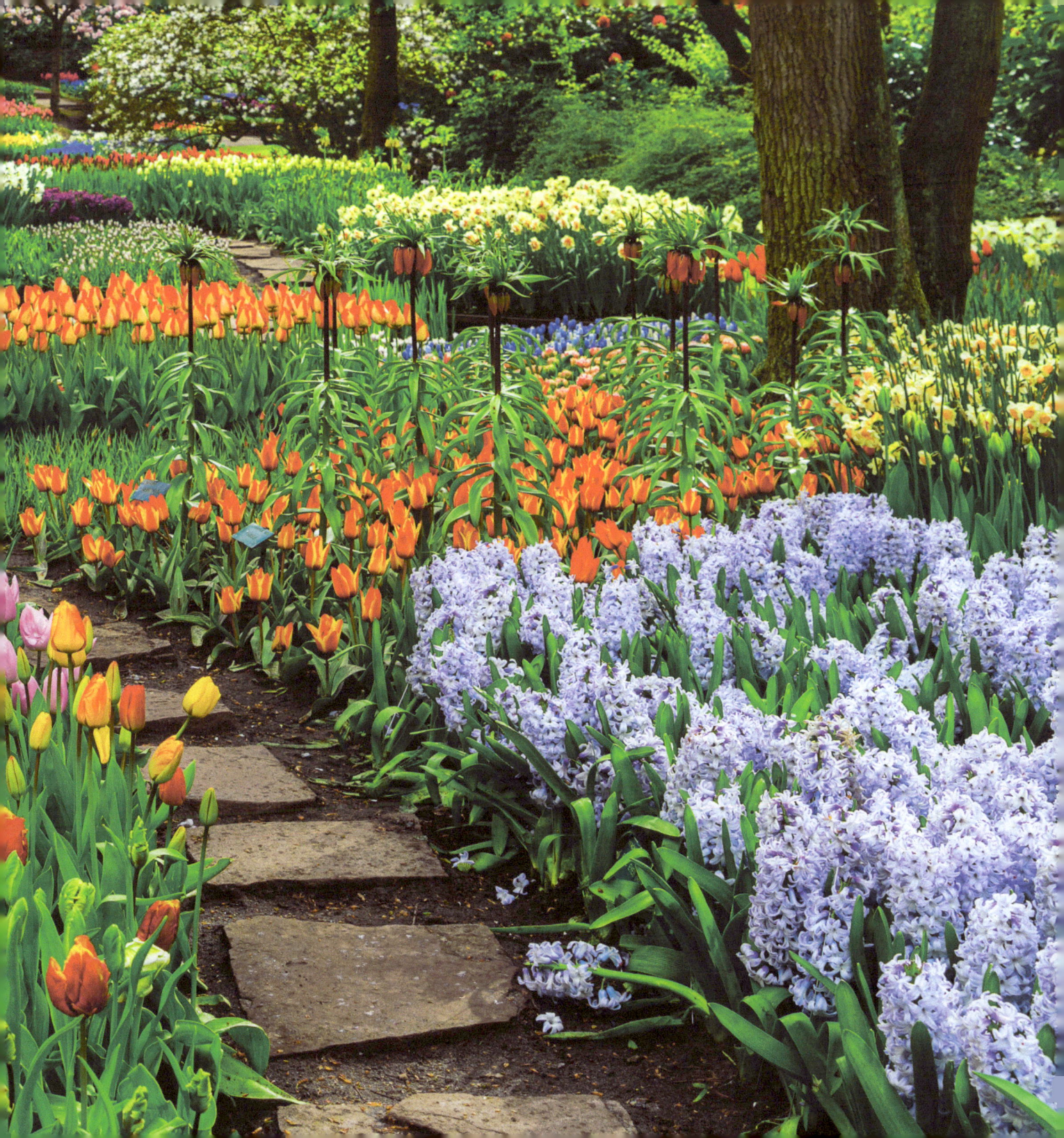

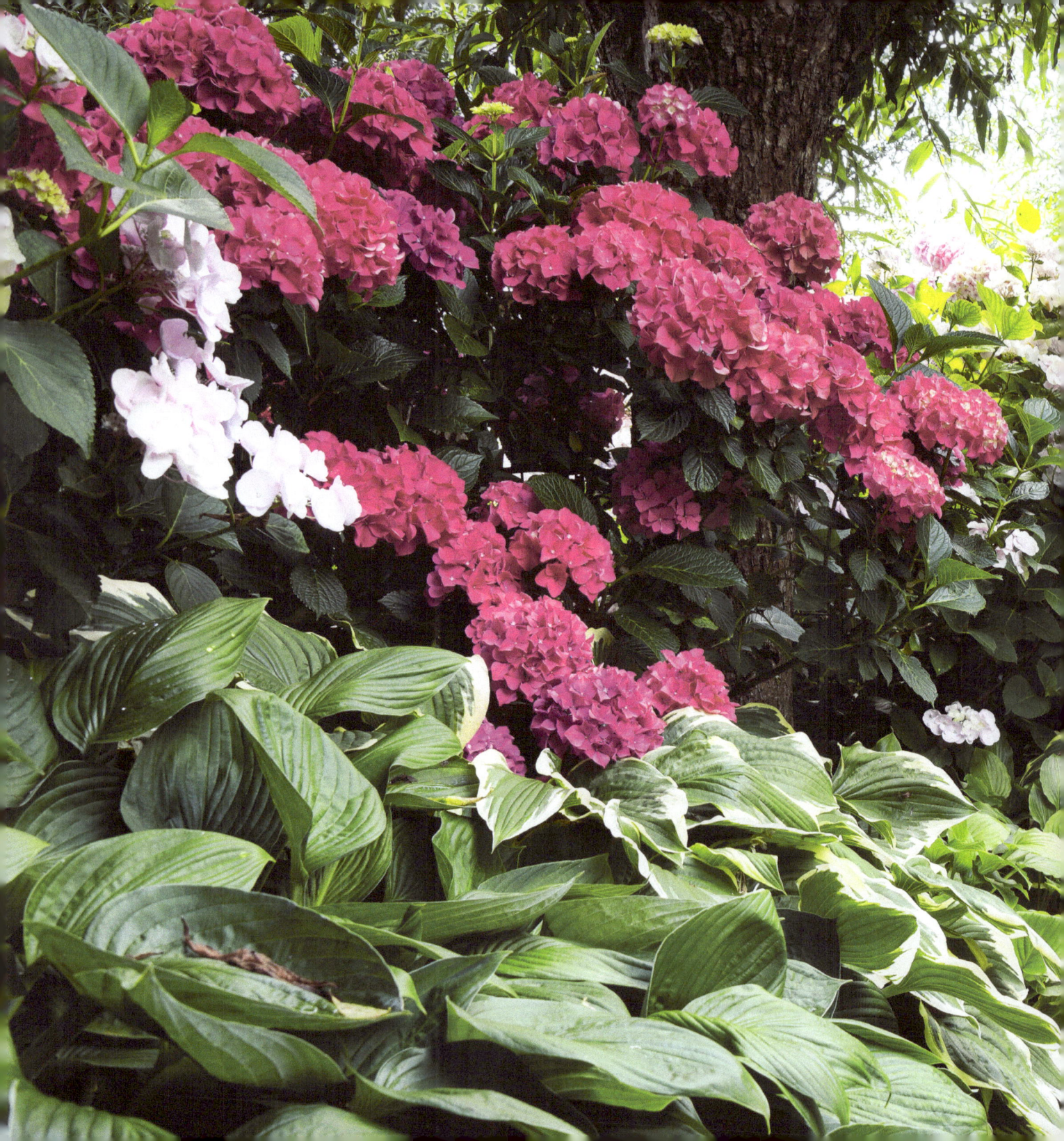

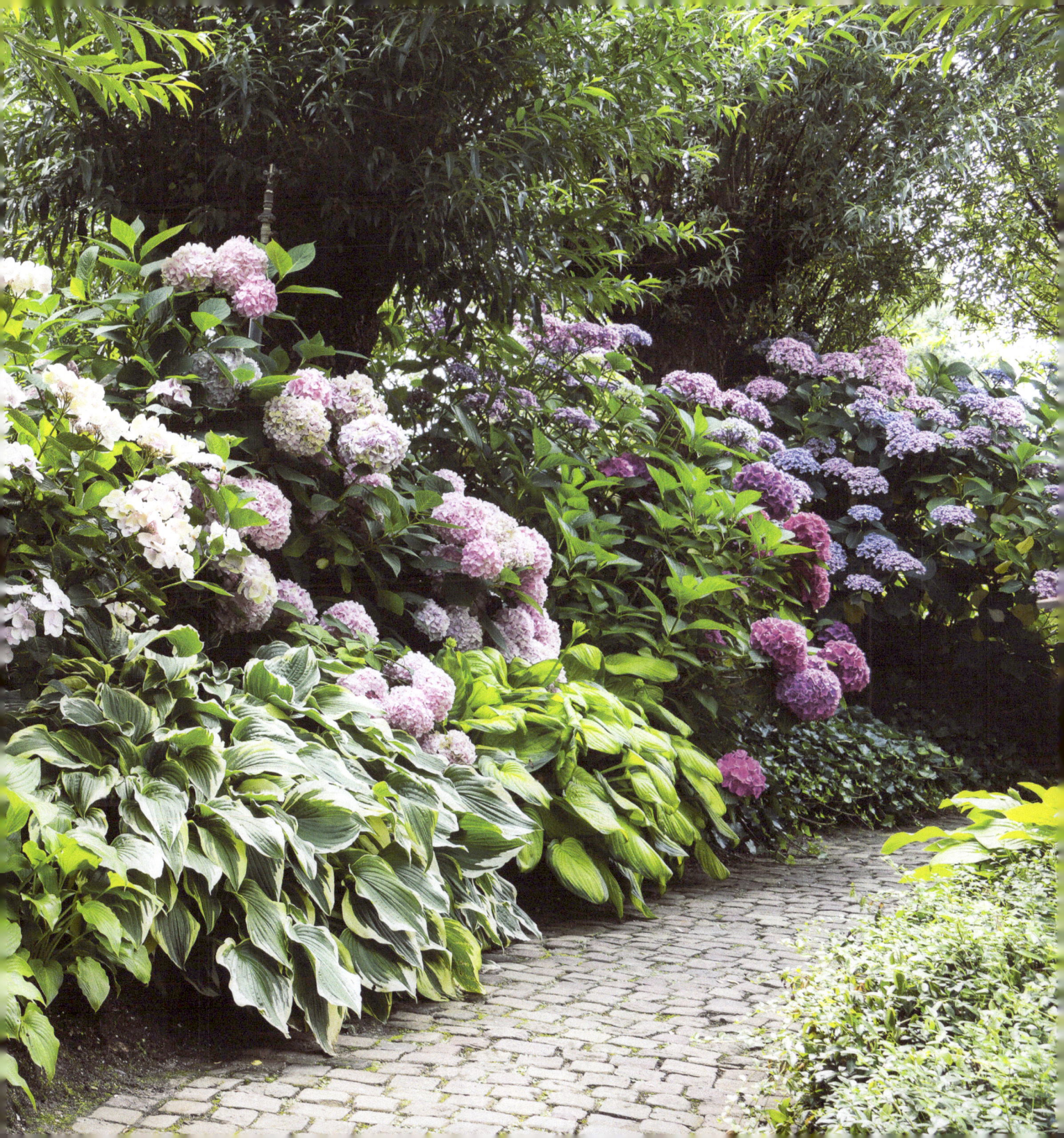

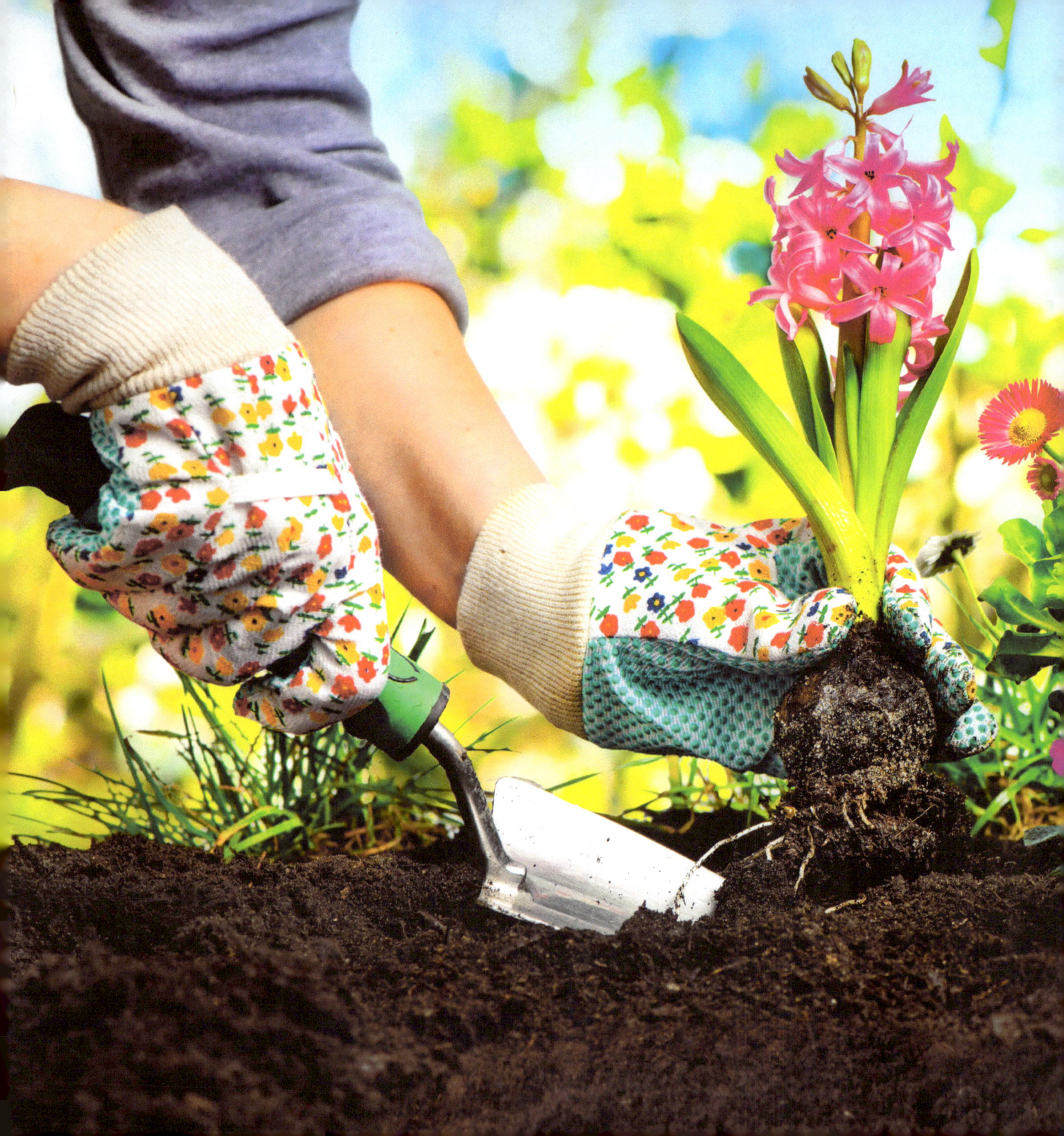

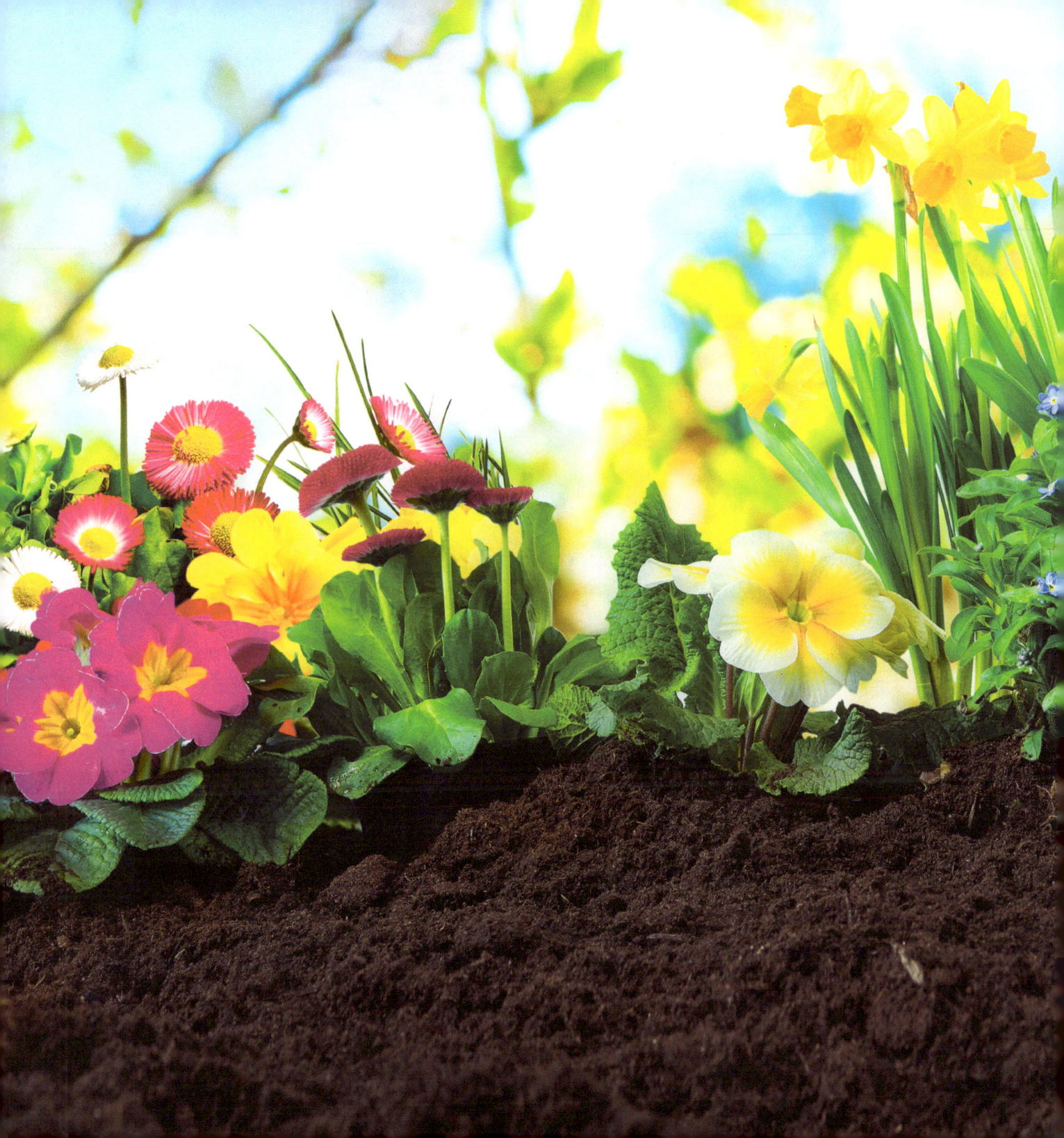

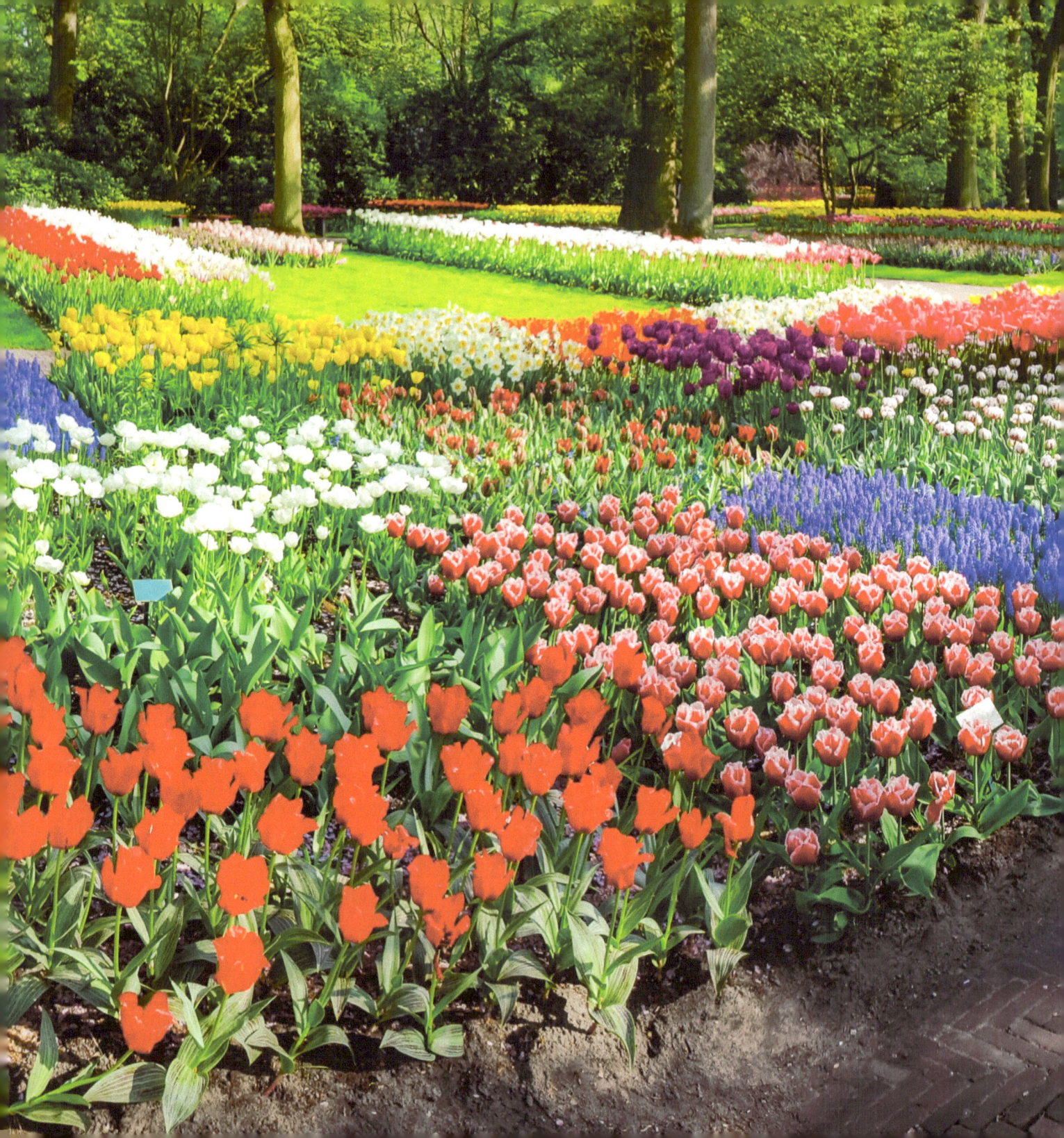

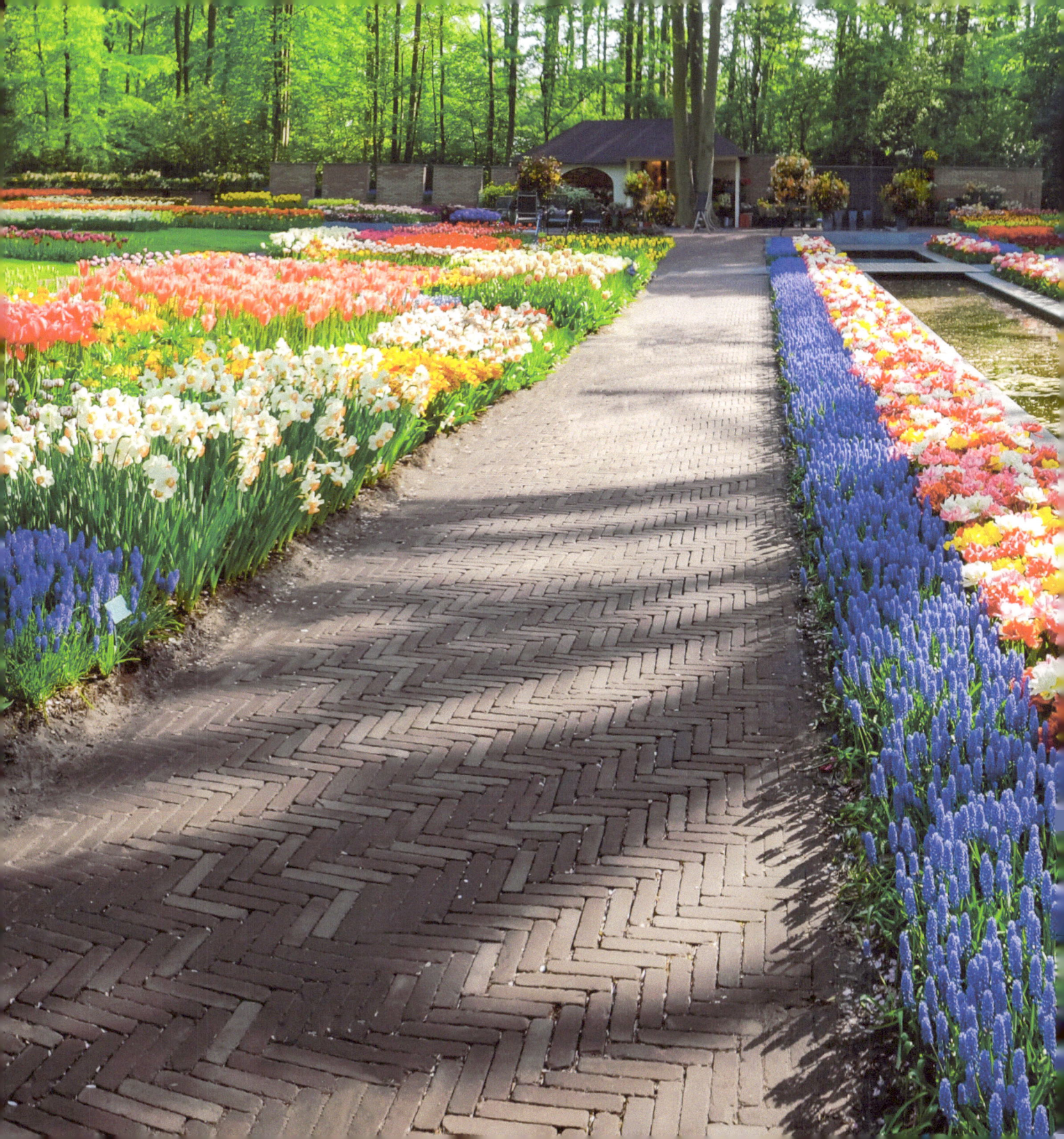

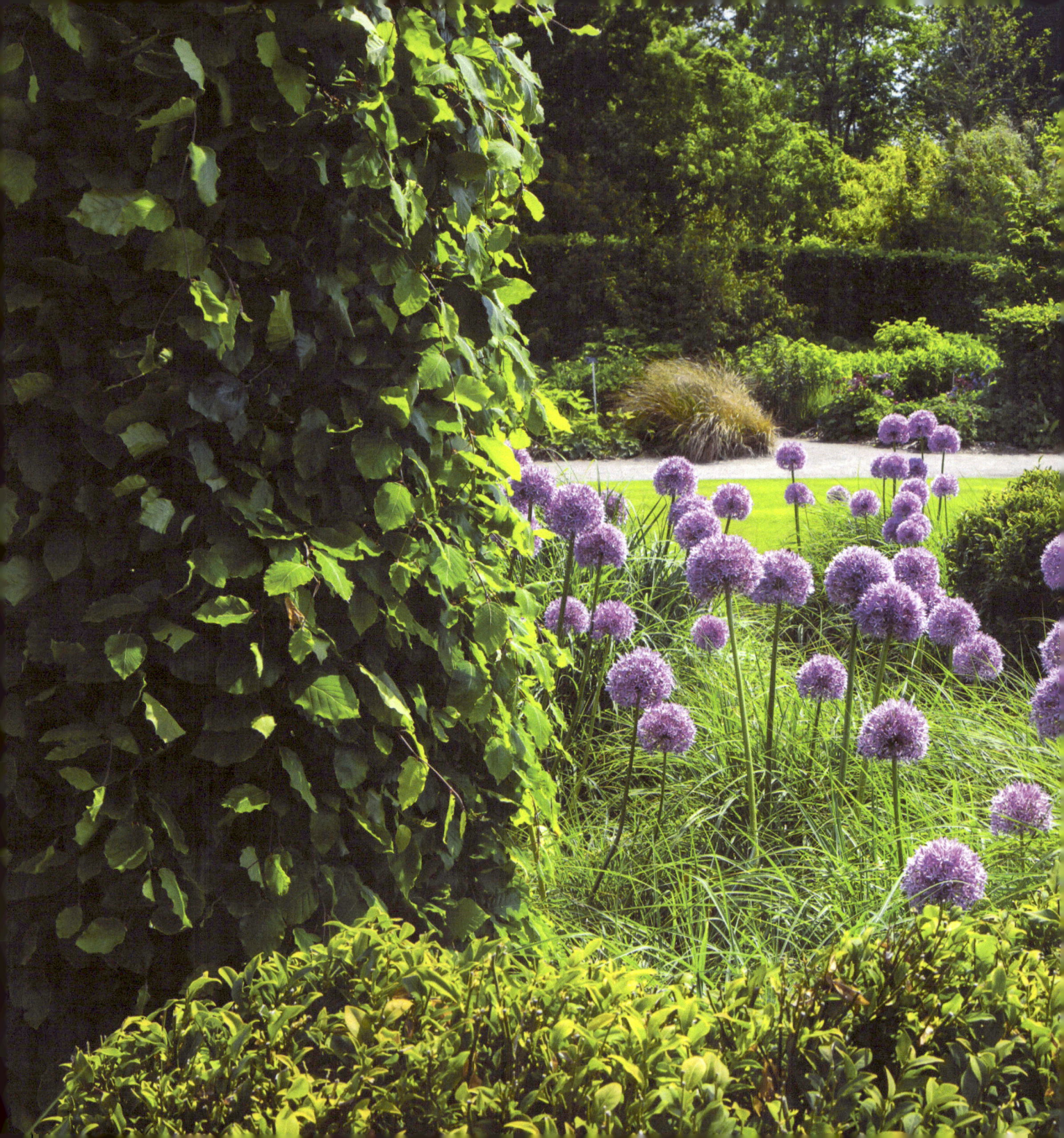

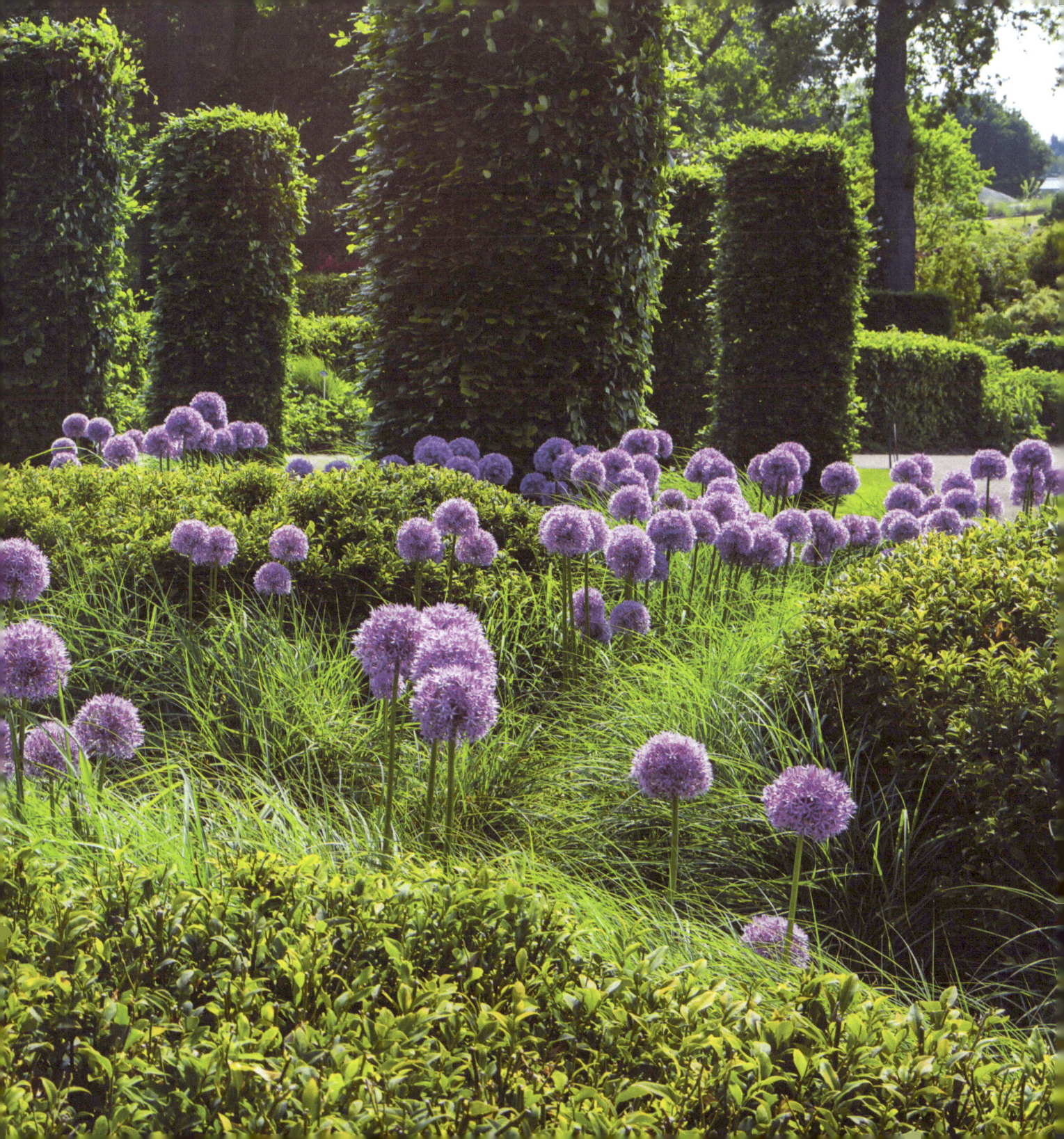

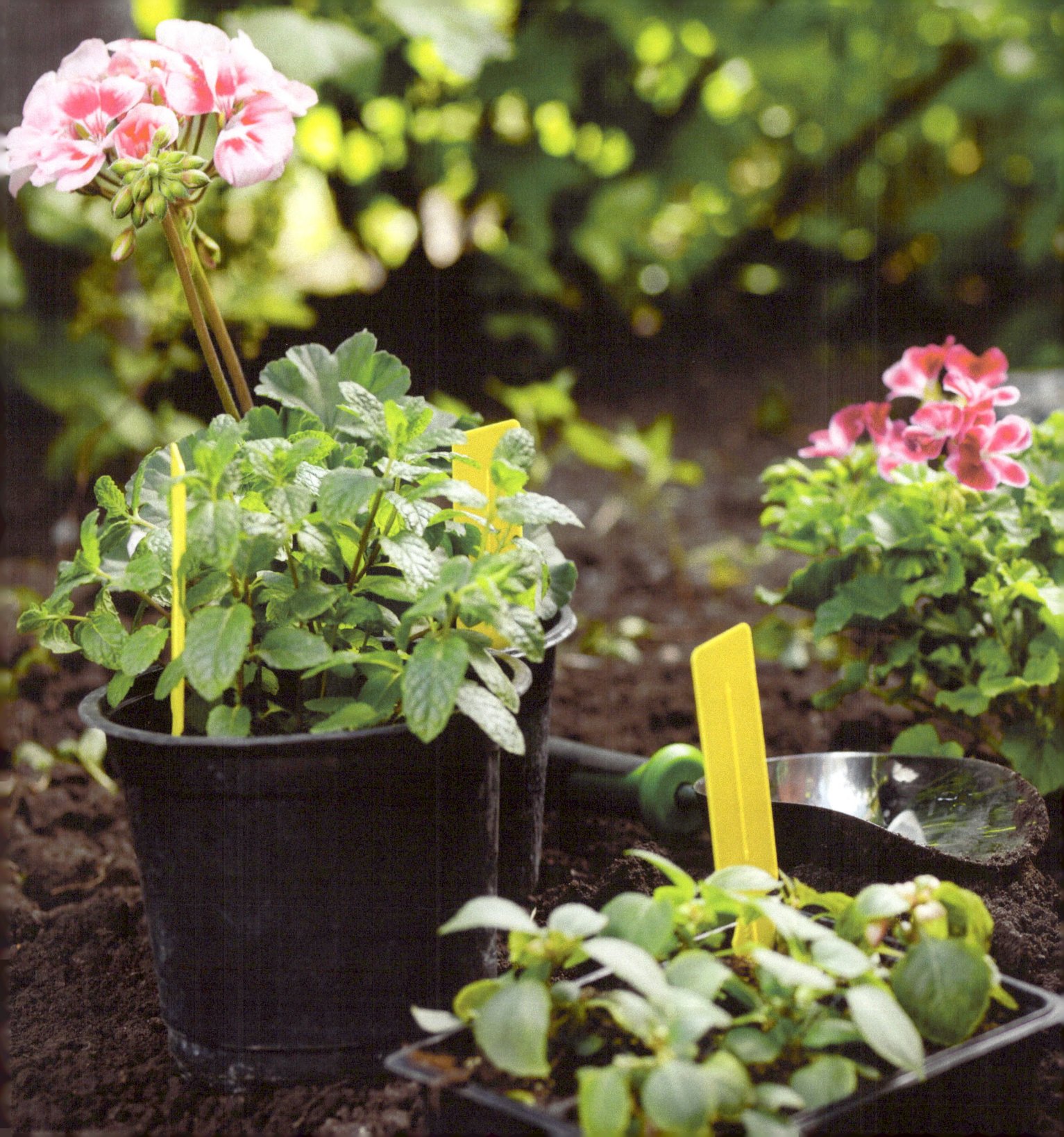

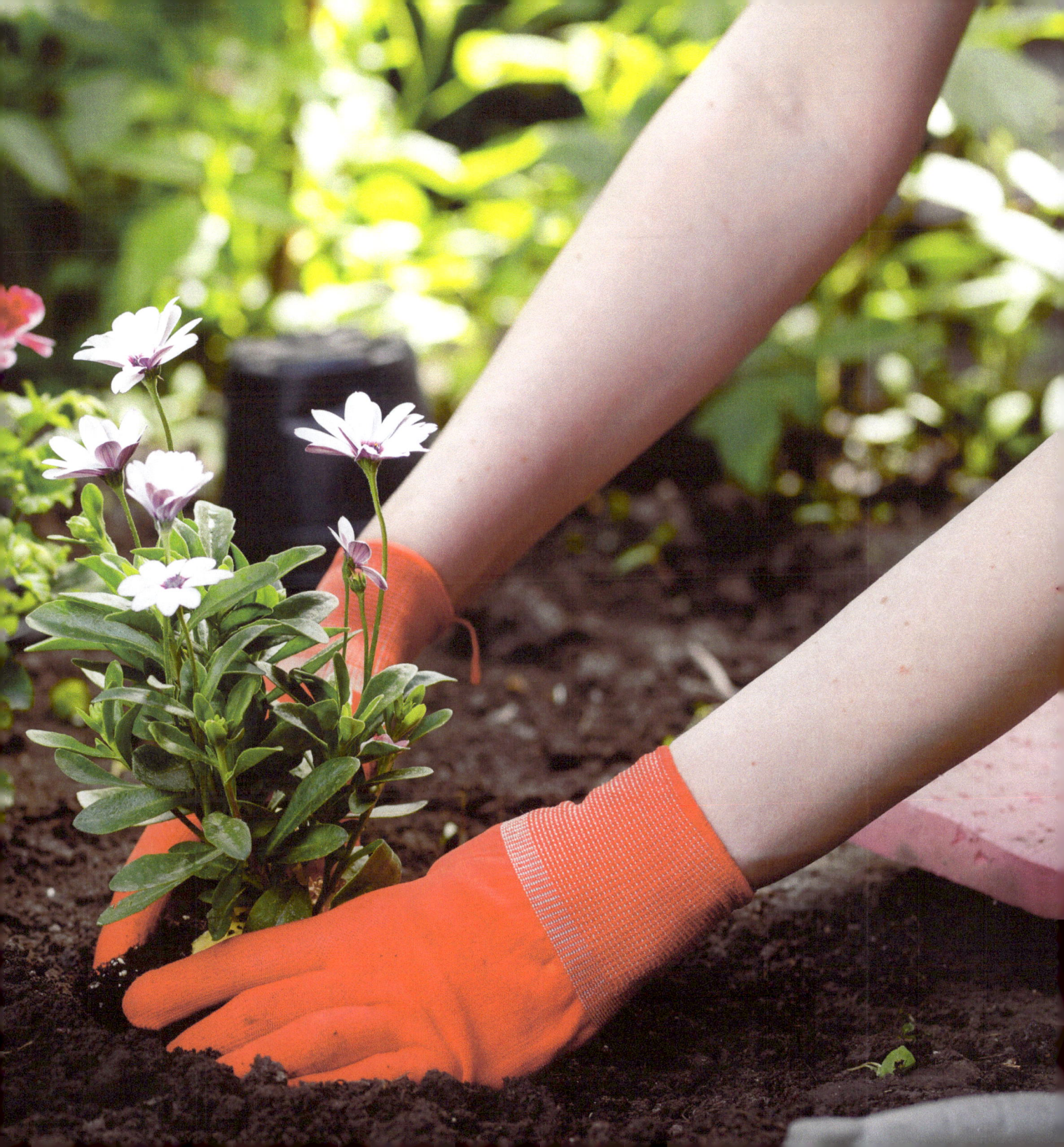

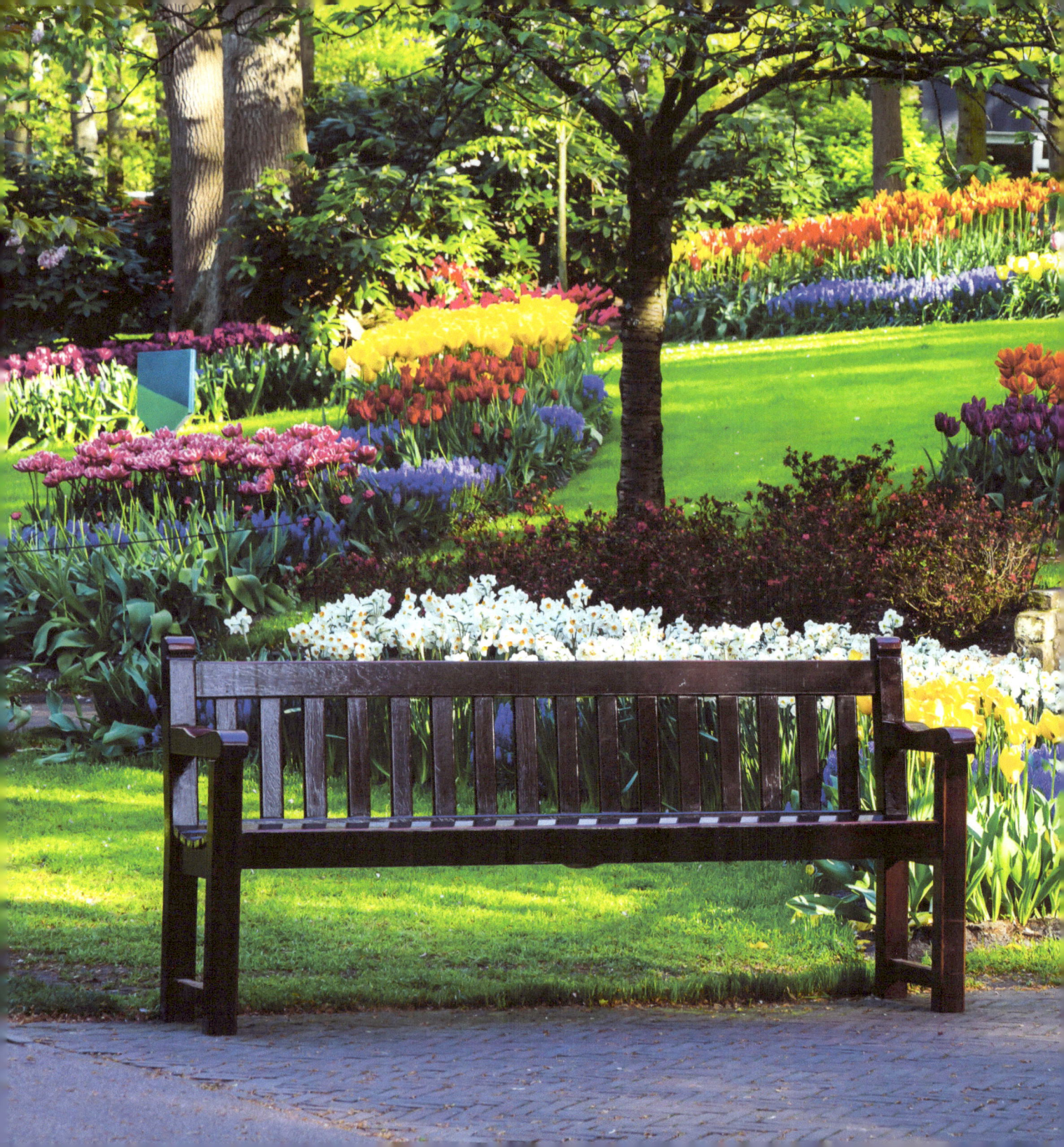

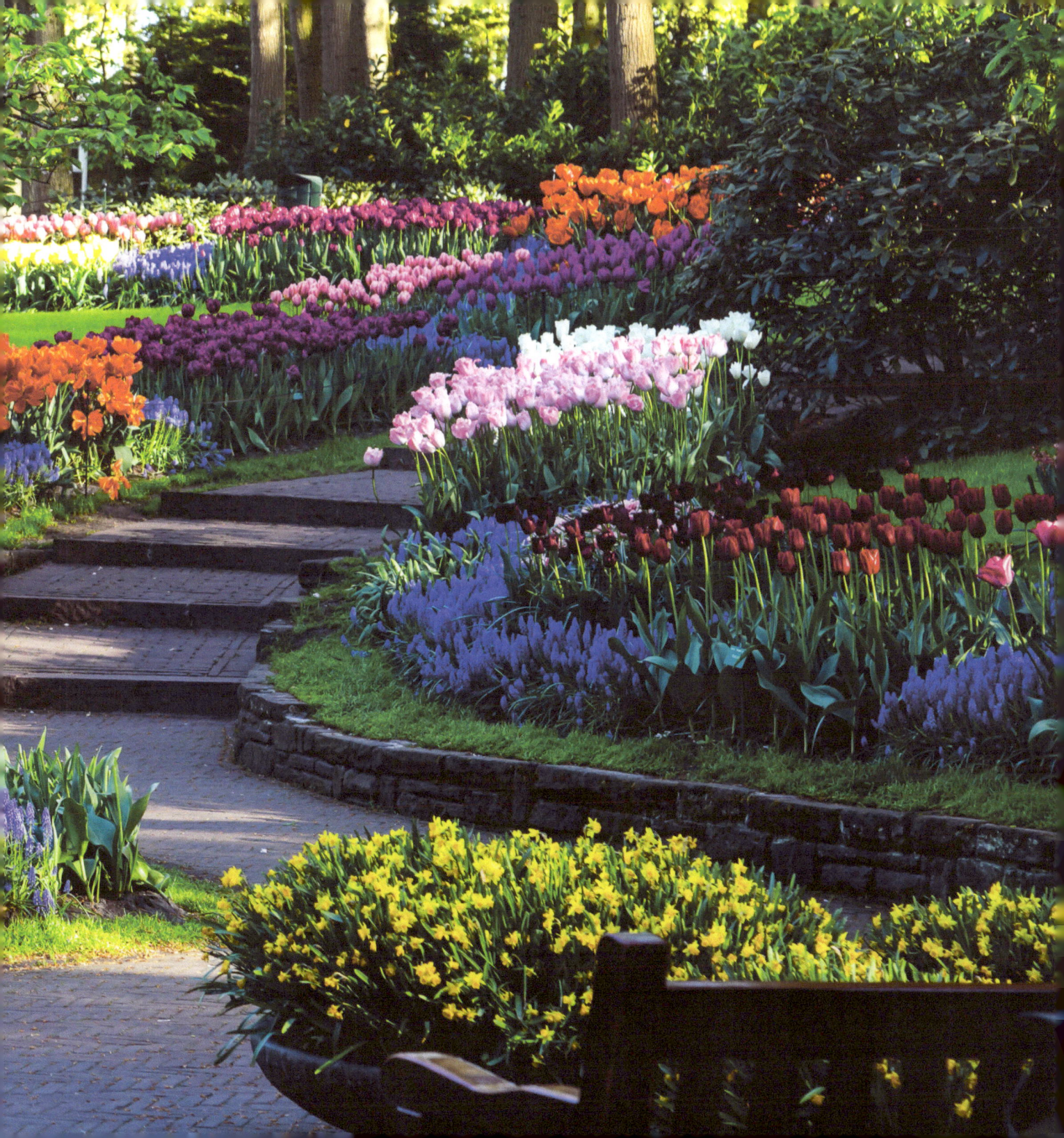

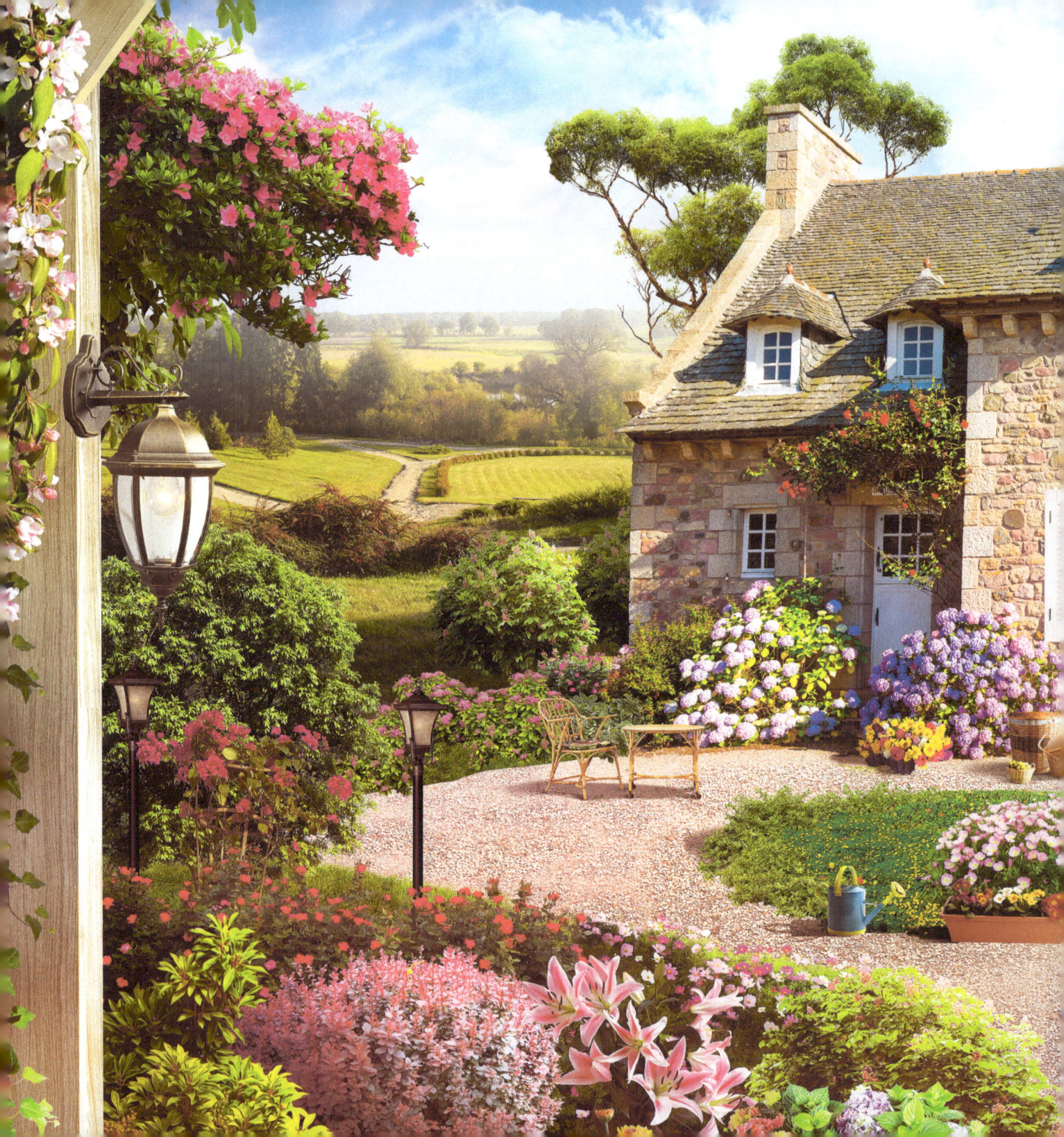

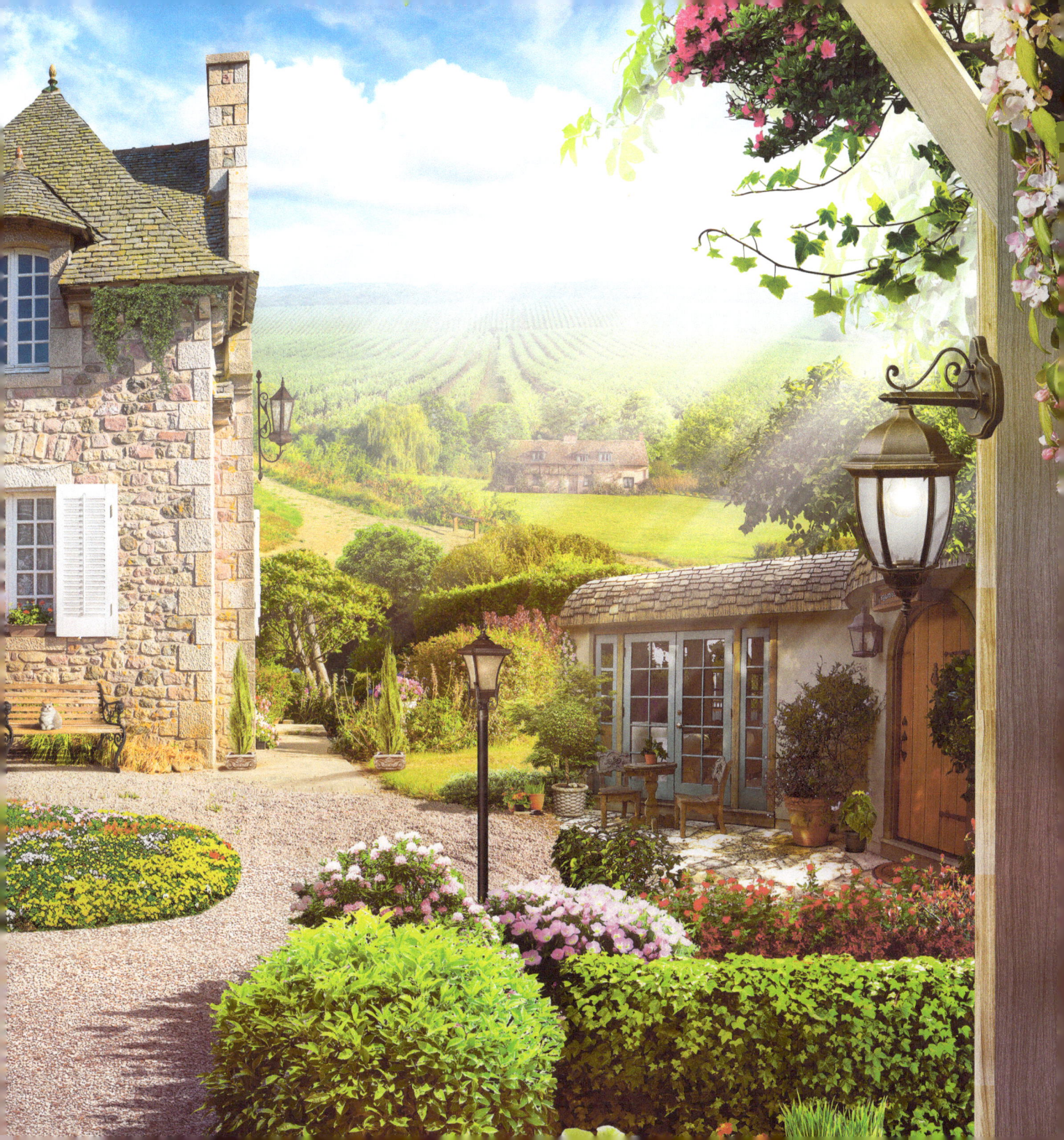

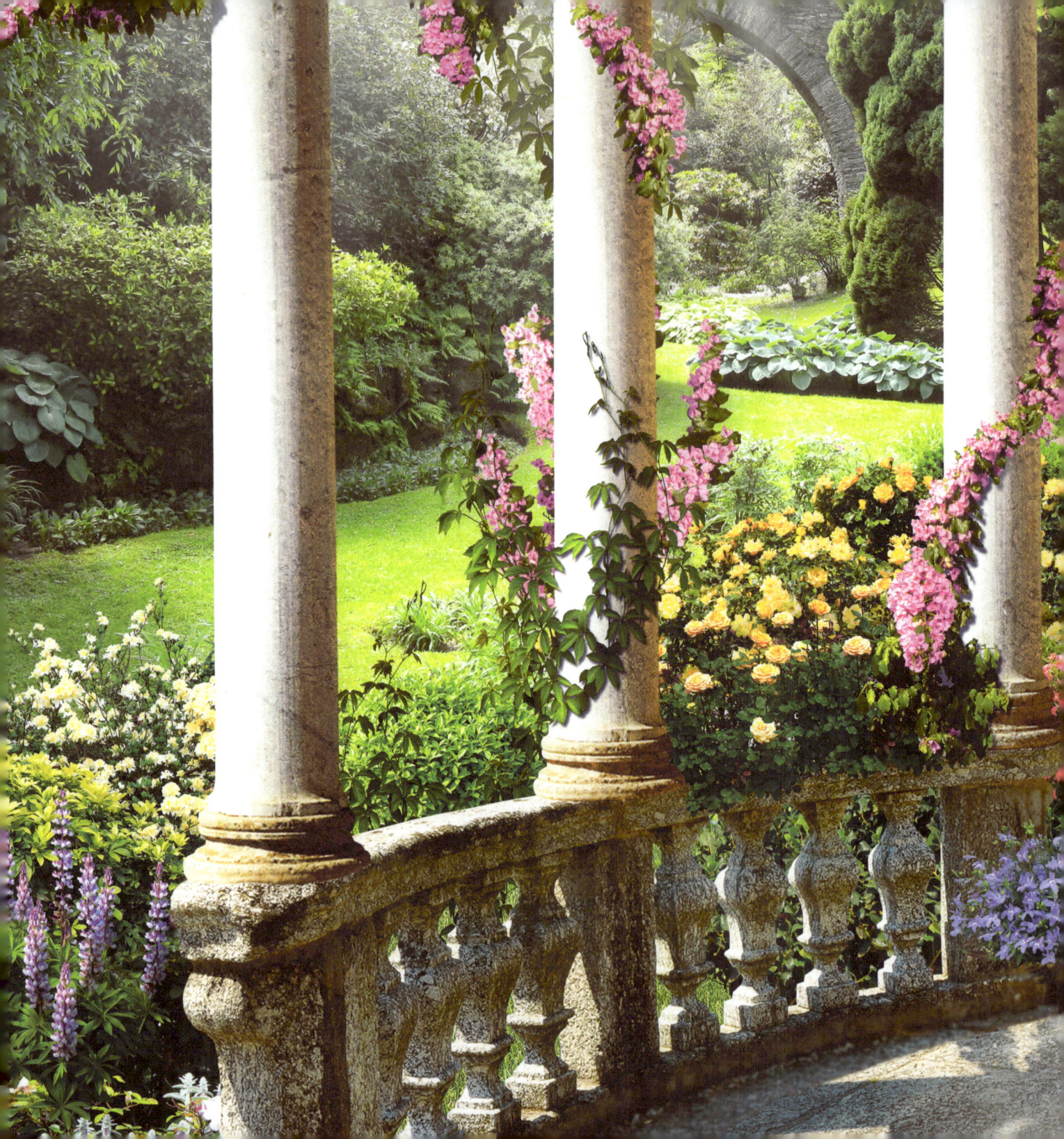

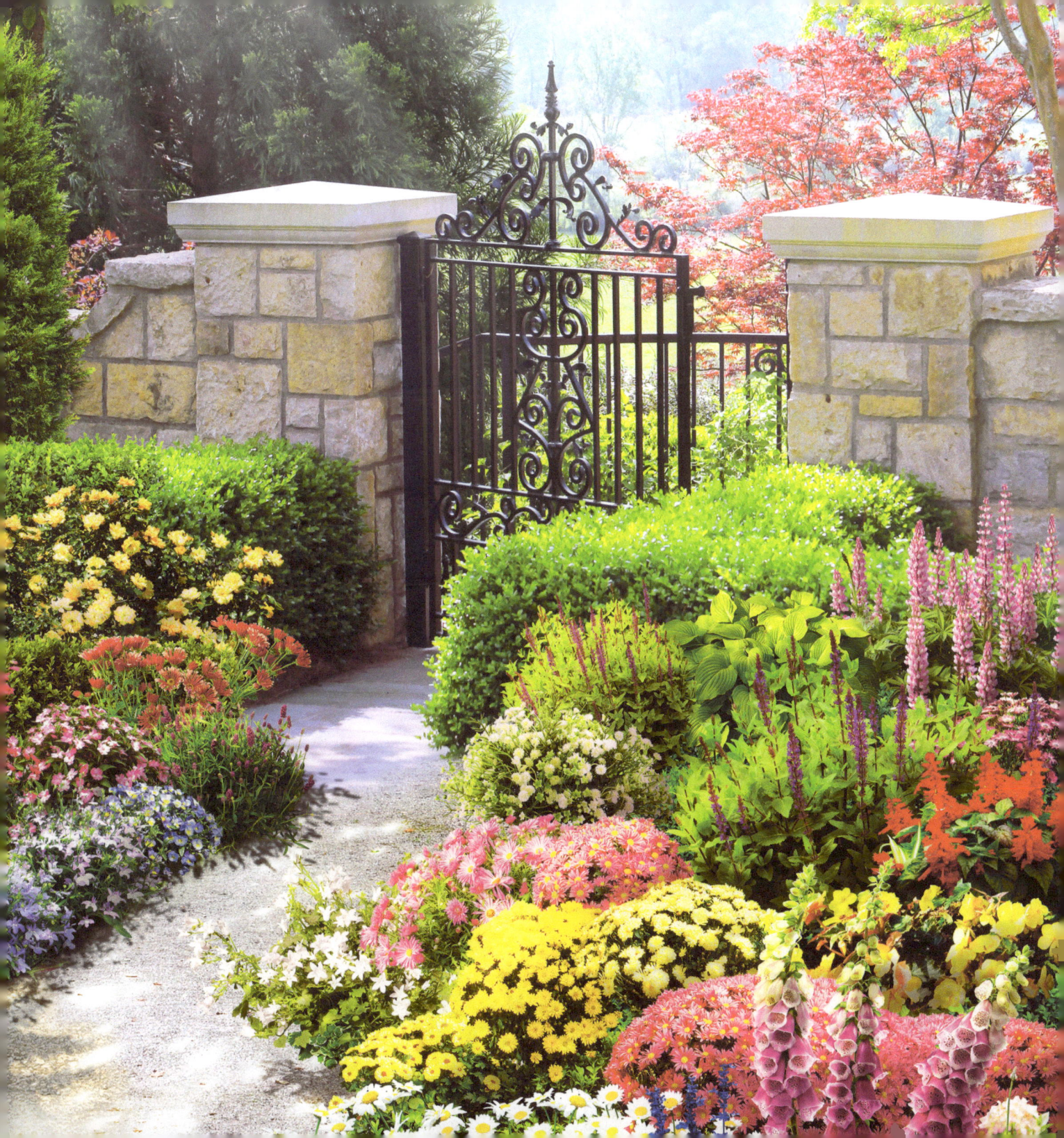

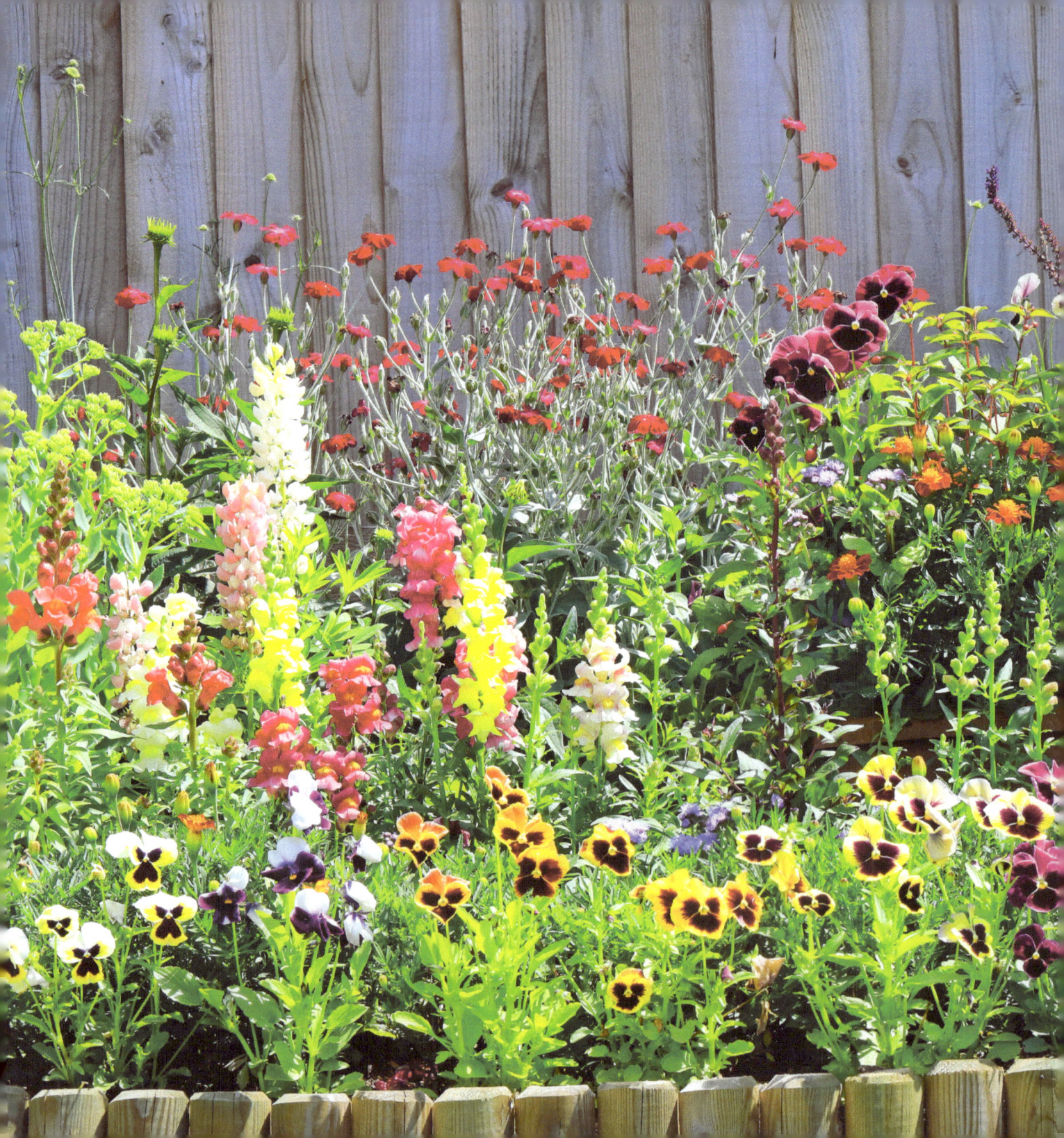

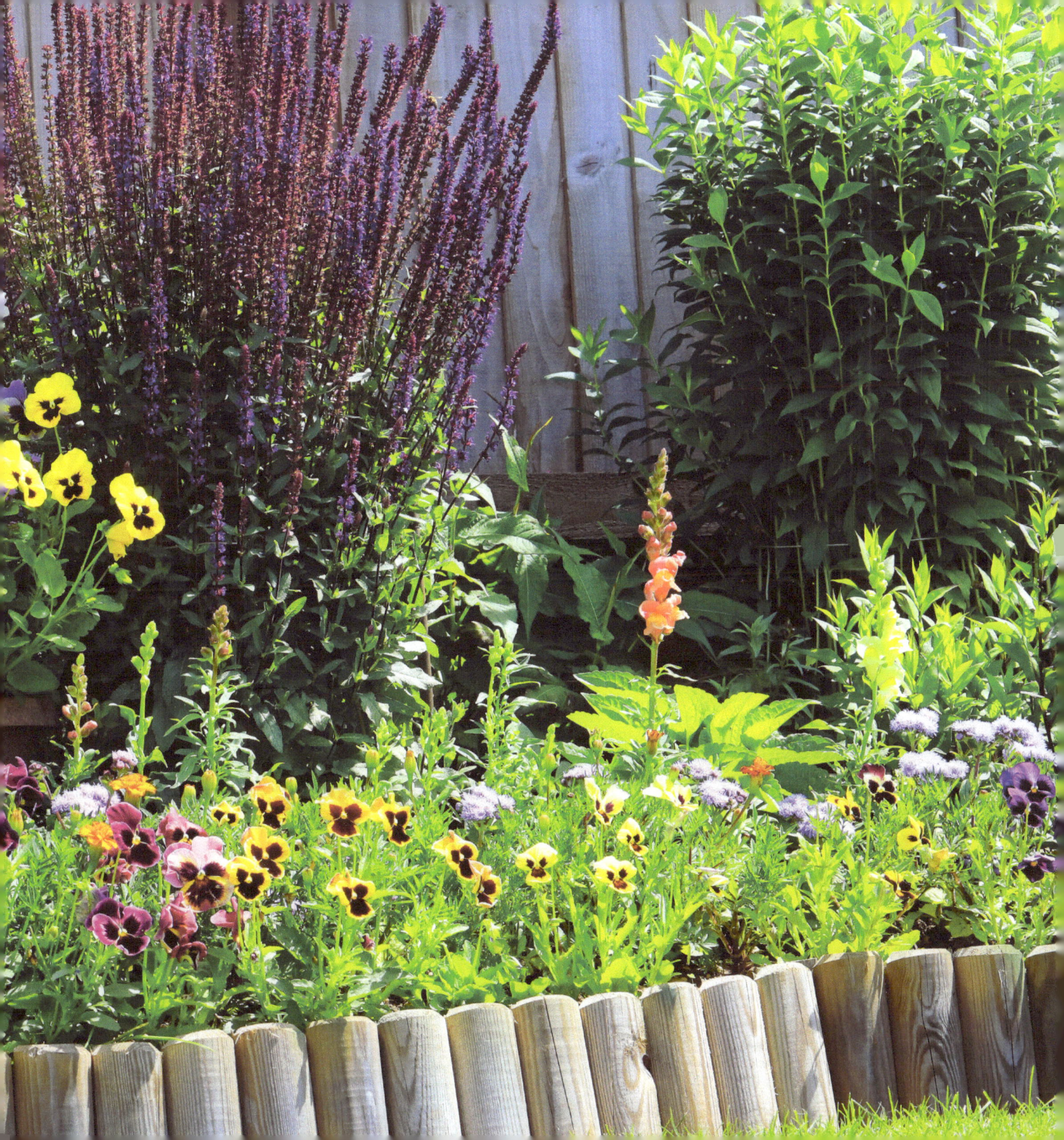

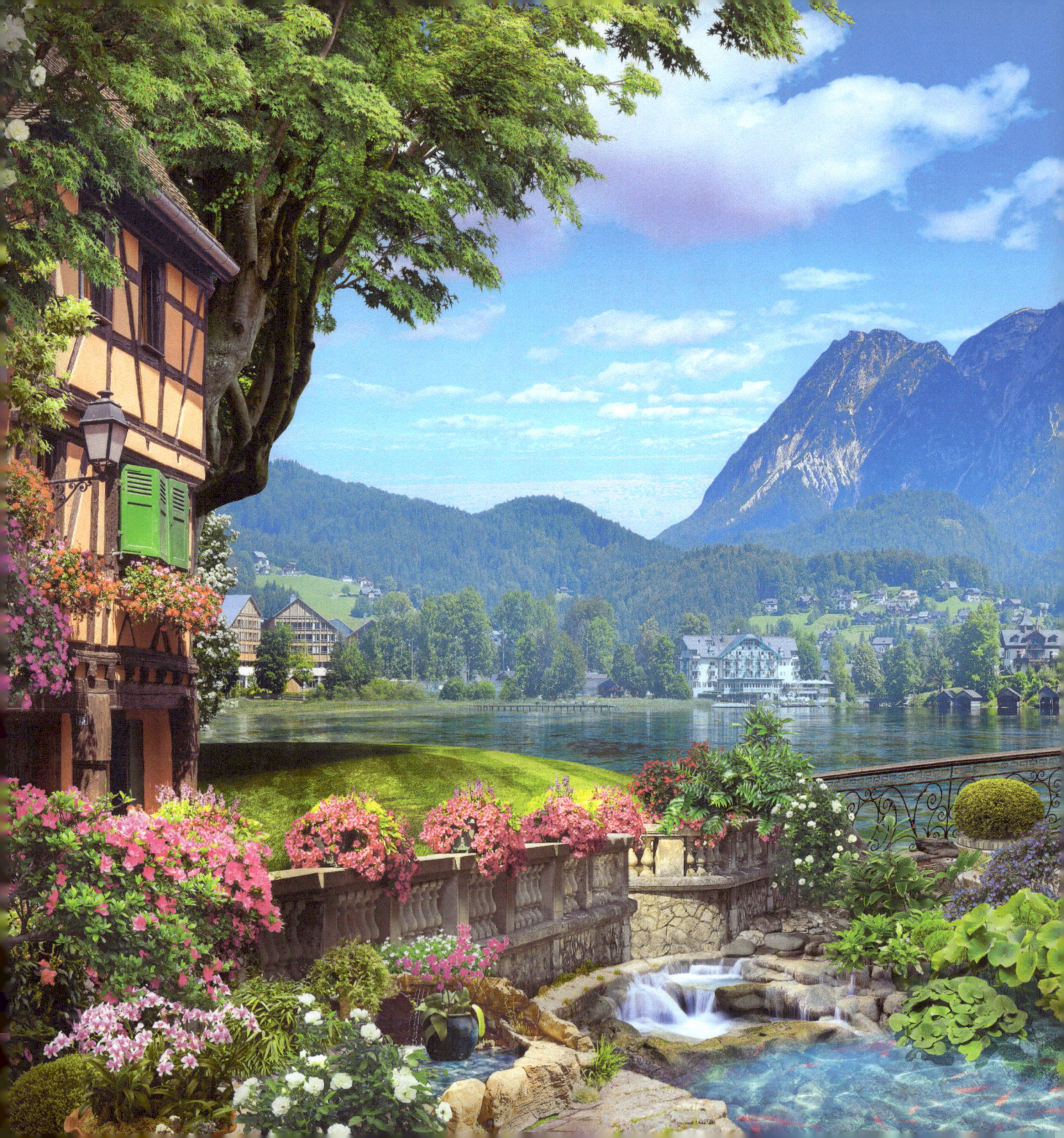

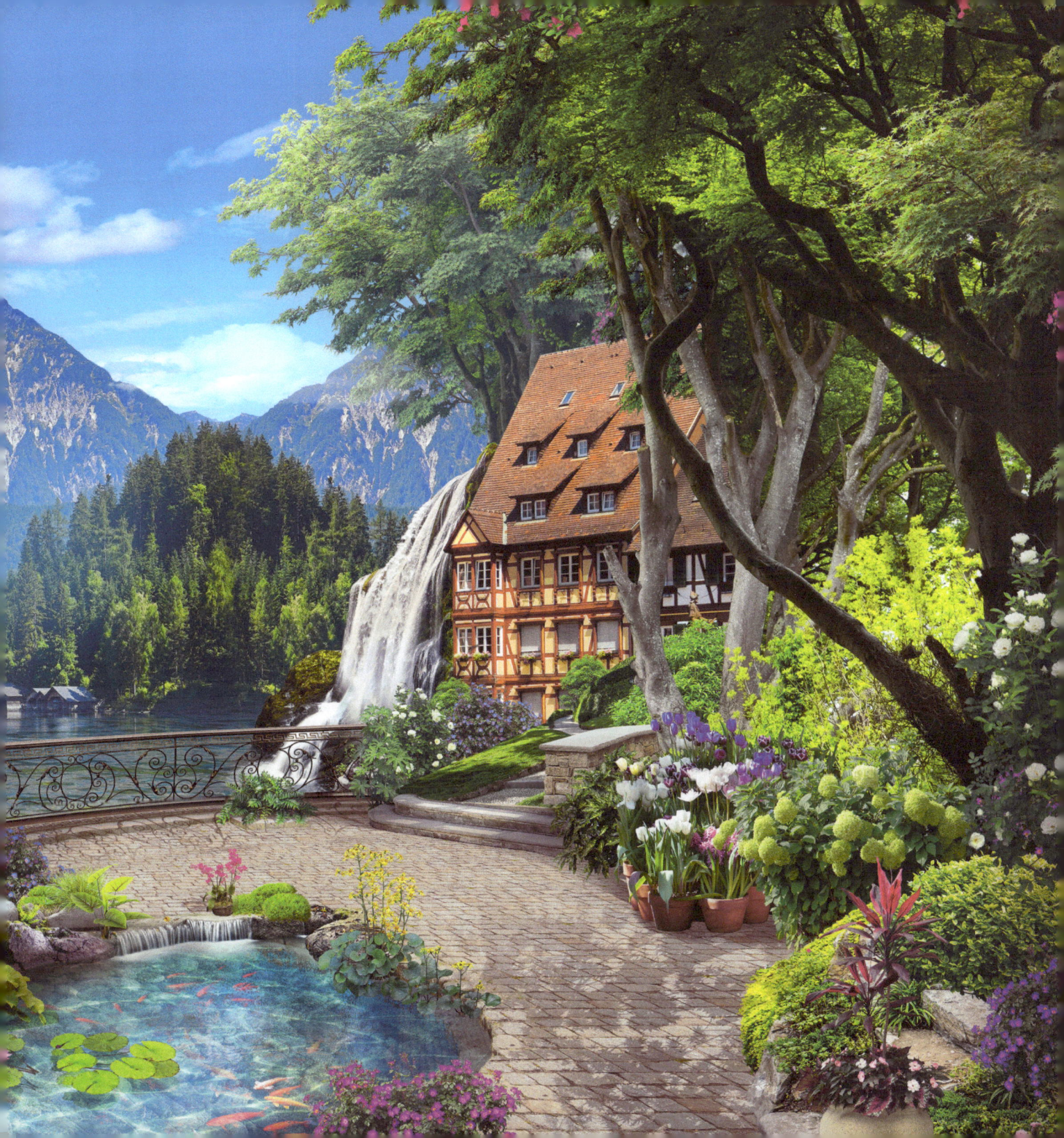

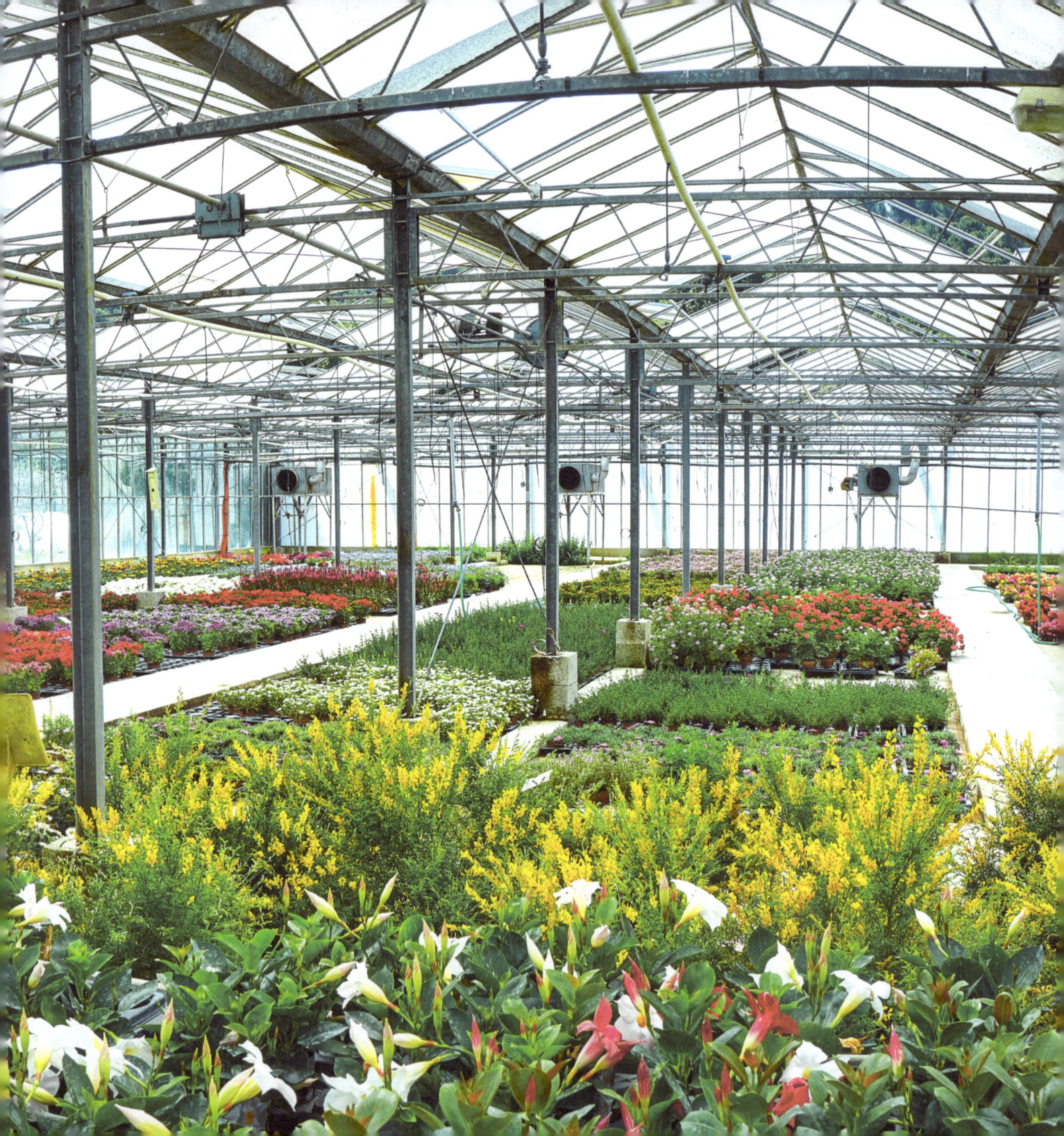

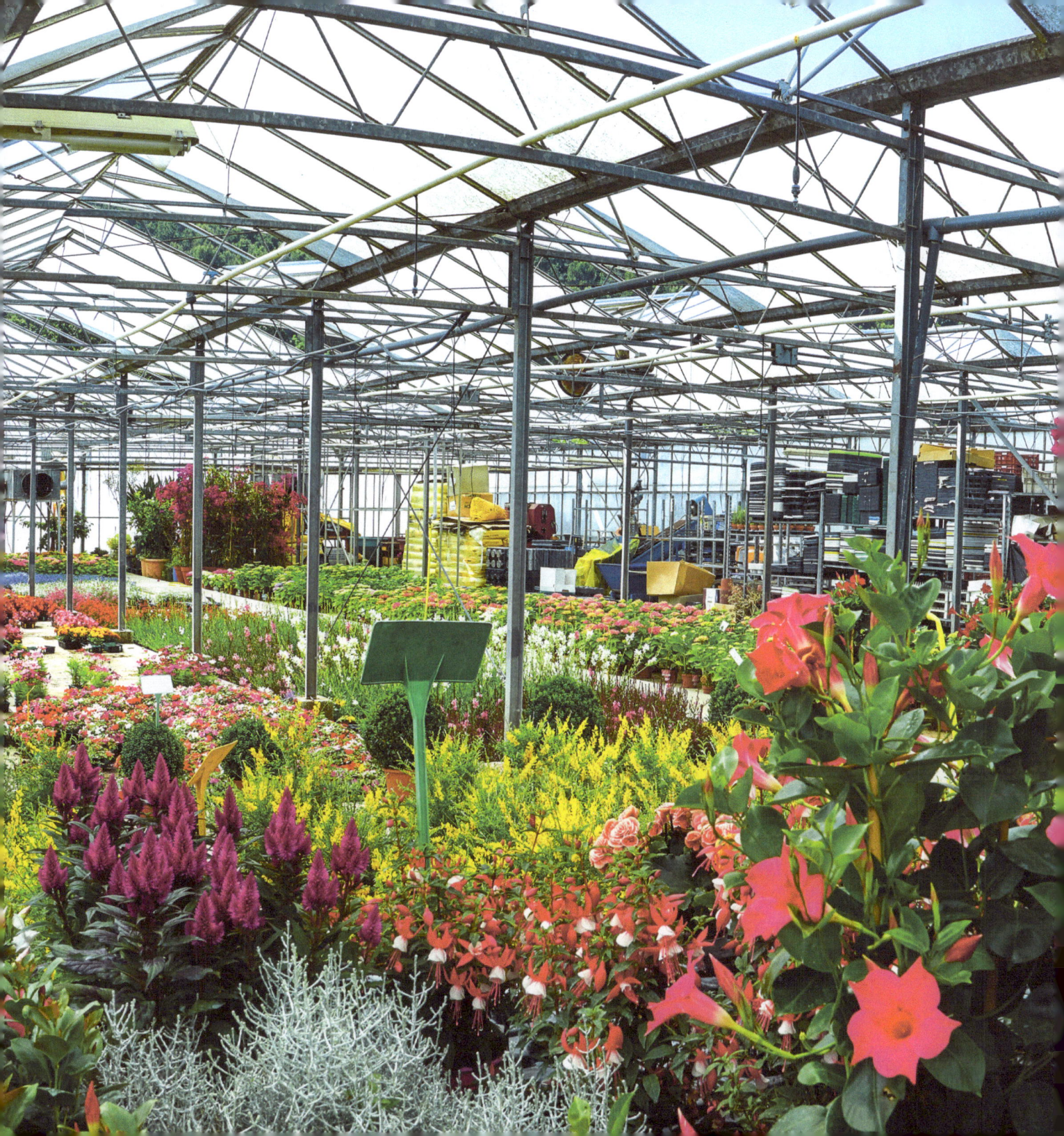

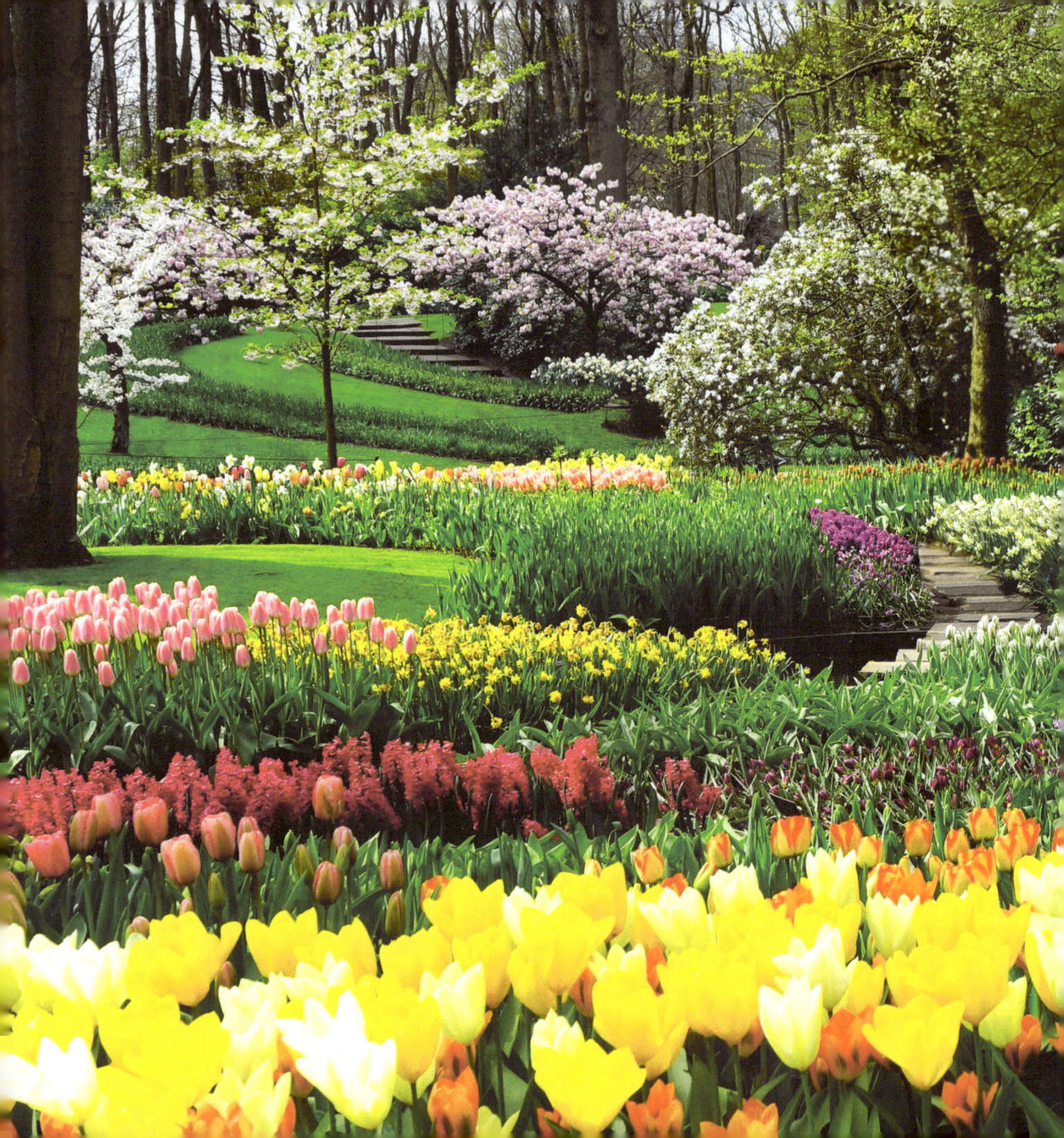

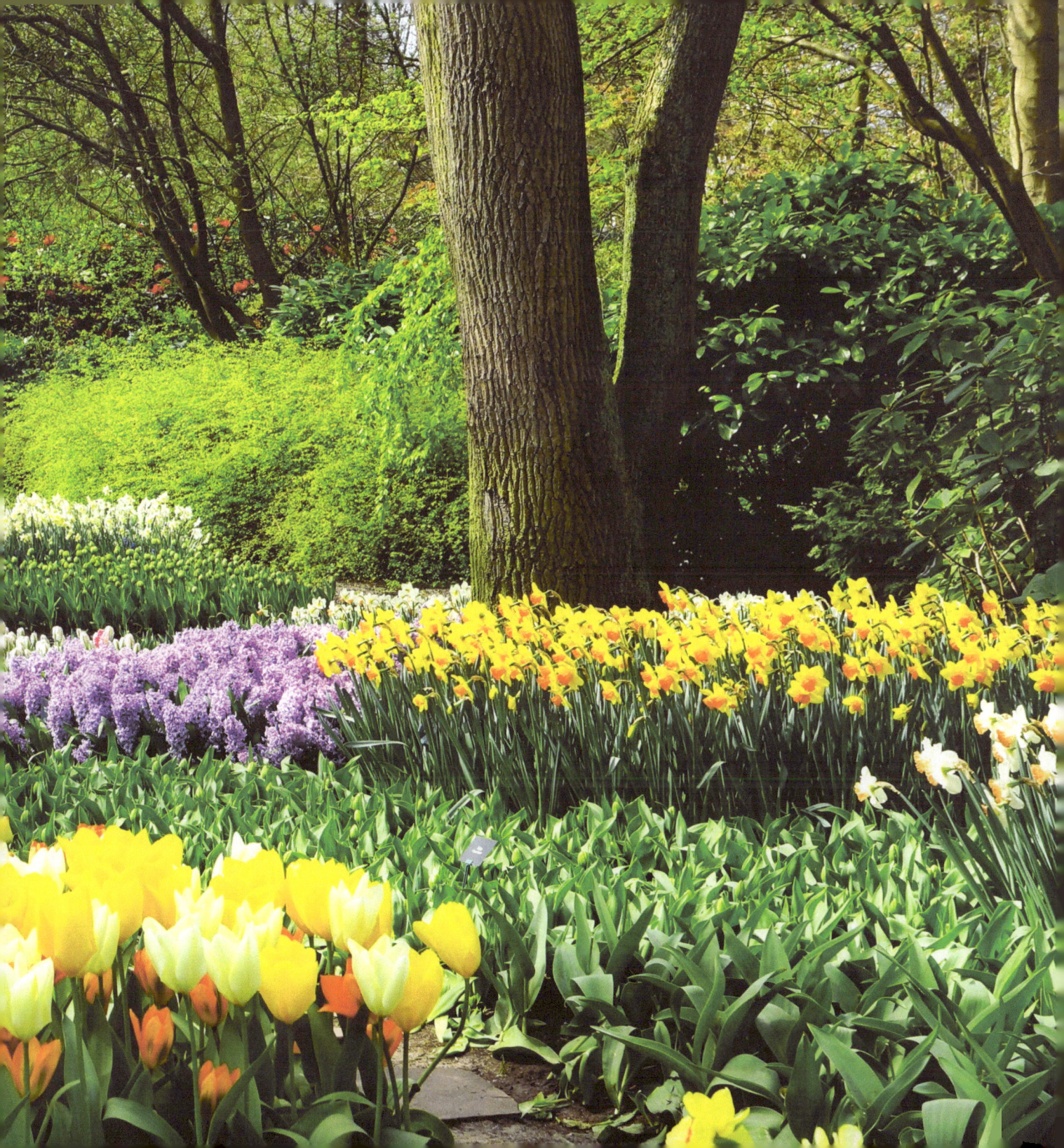

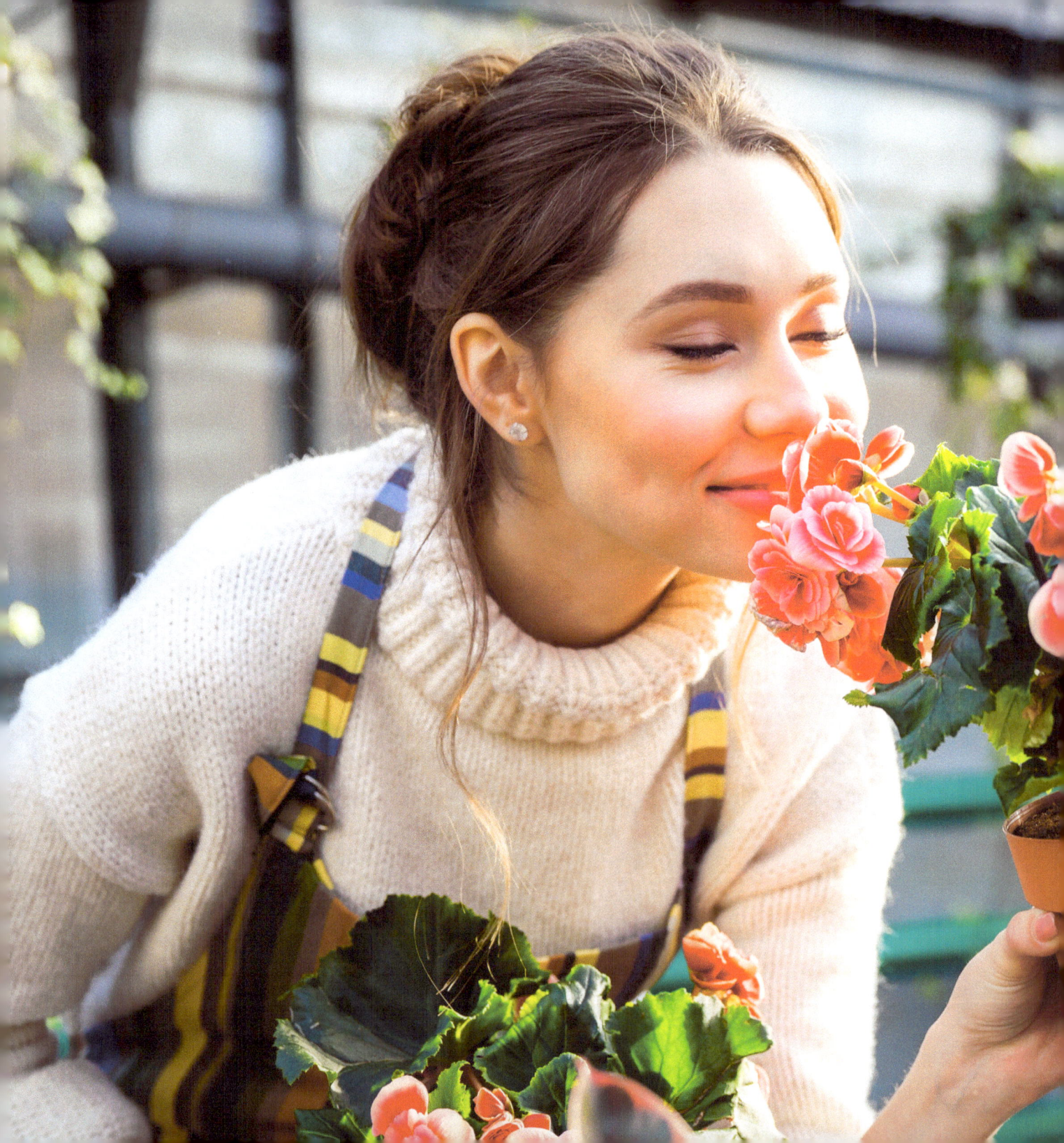

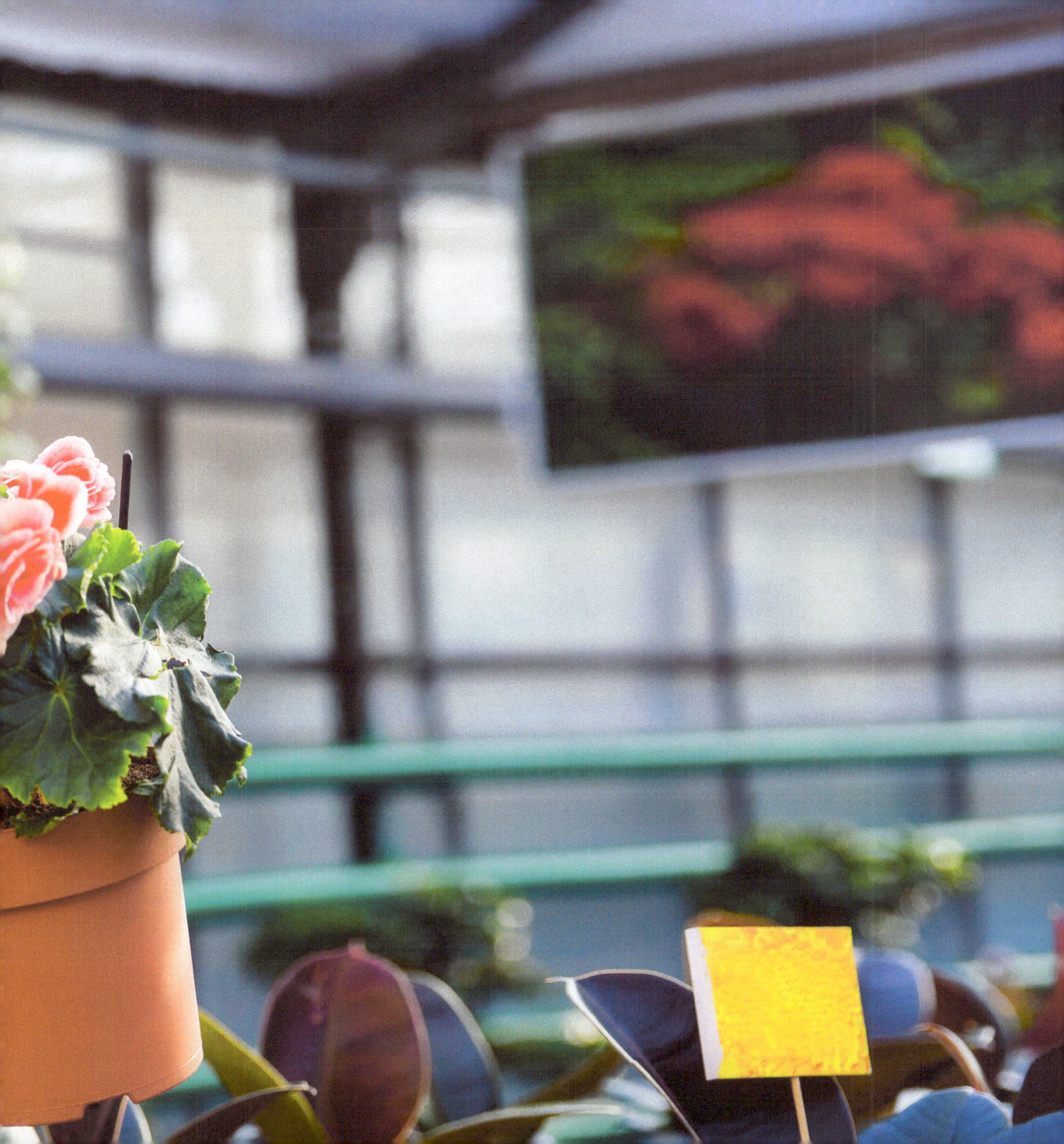

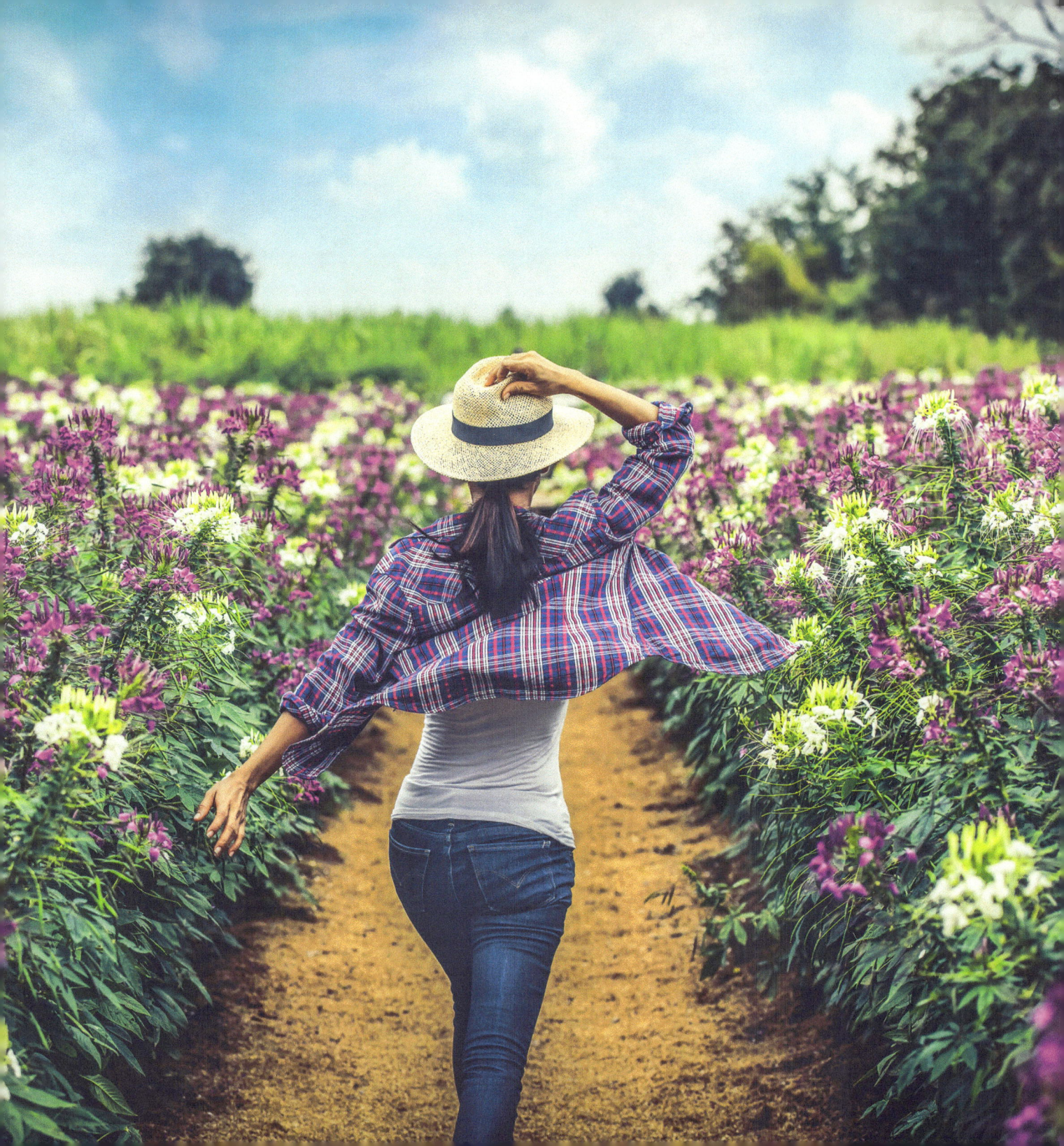

www.ingramcontent.com/pod-product-compliance
Lightning Source LLC
Chambersburg PA
CBHW061143030426
42335CB00002B/79